Sheffield Hallam University
Learning and IT Services
Collegiate Learning Centre
Collegiate Crescent Campus
Sheffield S10 2BP

101 870 636 4

D1586623

society, culture and health

an introduction to sociology for nurses

Karen Willis and Shandell Elmer

Sheffield Hallam University
Learning and Information Services
Withdrawn From Stock

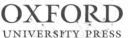

OXFORD
UNIVERSITY PRESS

OXFORD
UNIVERSITY PRESS

253 Normanby Road, South Melbourne, Victoria 3205, Australia

Oxford University Press is a department of the University of Oxford.
It furthers the University's objective of excellence in research,
scholarship, and education by publishing worldwide in

Oxford New York

Auckland Cape Town Dar es Salaam Hong Kong Karachi
Kuala Lumpur Madrid Melbourne Mexico City Nairobi
New Delhi Shanghai Taipei Toronto

With offices in

Argentina Austria Brazil Chile Czech Republic France Greece
Guatemala Hungary Italy Japan Poland Portugal Singapore
South Korea Switzerland Thailand Turkey Ukraine Vietnam

OXFORD is a trademark of Oxford University Press
in the UK and in certain other countries

Copyright © Karen Willis and Shandell Elmer 2007
First published 2007

Reproduction and communication for educational purposes
The Australian *Copyright Act 1968* (the Act) allows a maximum of one chapter
or 10% of the pages of this work, whichever is the greater, to be reproduced
and/or communicated by any educational institution for its educational purposes
provided that the educational institution (or the body that administers it) has
given a remuneration notice to Copyright Agency Limited (CAL) under the Act.

For details of the CAL licence for educational institutions contact:

Copyright Agency Limited
Level 19, 157 Liverpool Street
Sydney NSW 2000
Telephone: (02) 9394 7600
Facsimile: (02) 9394 7601
E-mail: info@copyright.com.au

Reproduction and communication for other purposes
Except as permitted under the Act (for example, any fair dealing
for the purposes of study, research, criticism or review) no part of this
book may be reproduced, stored in a retrieval system, communicated or
transmitted in any form or by any means without prior written permission.
All enquiries should be made to the publisher at the address above.

National Library of Australia Cataloguing-in-Publication data

Willis, Karen.
Society, culture and health : an introduction to sociology for nurses.

Bibliography.
Includes index.
ISBN 9780195559071 (pbk.).

1. Nursing—Social aspects. 2. Sociology. 3. Social medicine. I. Elmer, Shandell. II. Title.
610.73

Cover design, text design and typeset by Kerry Cooke, eggplant communications
Proofread by Anne Mulvaney
Indexed by Jeanne Rudd
Printed in Hong Kong by Sheck Wah Tong Printing Press Ltd

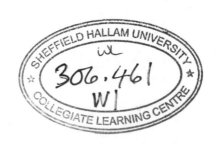

Contents

Guided tour

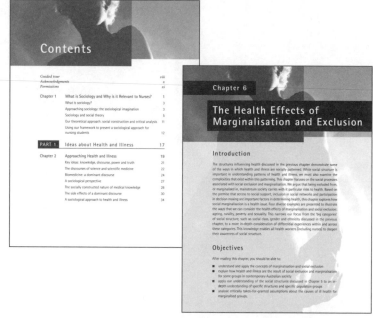

Society, Culture and Health explains how and why sociology is relevant to nursing

Objectives at the start of each chapter identify the key issues and concepts that will be covered in the chapter

Case studies throughout the book invite analysis about sociological issues related to either a specific illness or a nursing approach to a particular state of well-being. Each case study is followed by a set of questions.

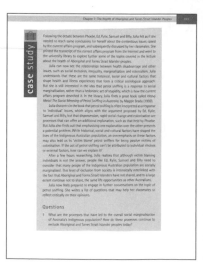

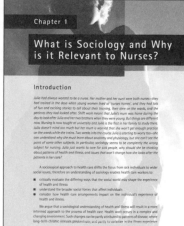

Opening case revisited introduces 'Julia' to help readers identify with the experiences of student nurses, and to illustrate the impact of sociological issues and theories on nursing practice

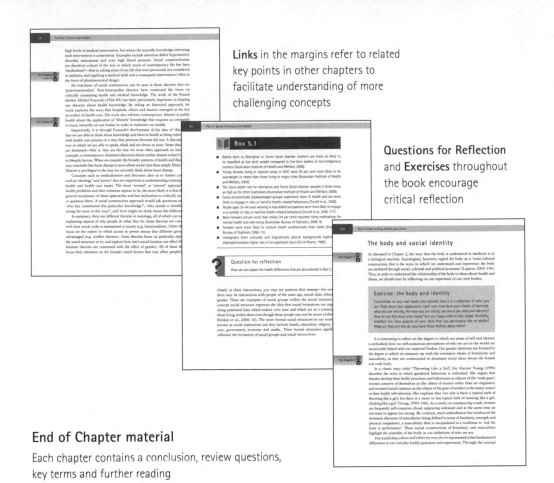

Links in the margins refer to related key points in other chapters to facilitate understanding of more challenging concepts

Questions for Reflection and **Exercises** throughout the book encourage critical reflection

End of Chapter material

Each chapter contains a conclusion, review questions, key terms and further reading

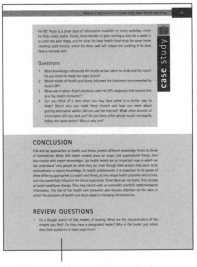

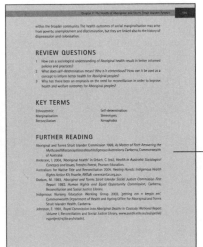

Review questions at the end of each chapter stimulate discussion and encourage critical thinking

Further Reading includes reference to useful websites, journal articles and reference books which are chosen for readability and accessibility

Acknowledgments

Karen and Shandell would like to thank Professor Rob White for his encouragement to embark on this endeavour. We are also deeply appreciative of the support and assistance provided by Kellie Brandenburg and Melody West in locating and preparing case studies and examples. We have also enjoyed the support of our colleagues at the School of Sociology and Social Work and the Department of Rural Health at the University of Tasmania.

We are grateful for the advice and guidance that we have received from the staff at Oxford University Press: Debra James provided enthusiasm and ongoing support for the project, along with Caitlin Matthews and Tim Campbell. Thanks also to the anonymous reviewers who provided us with insightful feedback.

We would both like to thank our family and friends. Shandell would particularly like to thank her family and friends for their belief in her ability and for their love and patience, which endured when tested. Karen wishes to thank her partner, Bengt, who always provides unconditional love and support.

Finally, we would like to acknowledge each other. In a world of constant deadlines and pressures to produce, we have maintained and strengthened our friendship.

Permissions

The following organisations and institutions also kindly agreed to give permission to reproduce or adapt material, and their assistance and cooperation is gratefully acknowledged.

The organisation *Australians for Native Title and Reconciliation* (ANTaR) is thanked for permission to reproduce ANTaR's Indigenous Health Rights Statement <http://www.antar.org.au>.

The *Australian Bureau of Statistics* is thanked for permission to present material from the following sources: Australian Bureau of Statistics 2006, *National Health Survey Summary of Results, 2004–2005*, Catalogue No. 4364.0, Australian Bureau of Statistics, Canberra, ABS data used with permission from the Australian Bureau of Statistics; Australian Bureau of Statistics 2004, *Year Book of Australia 2004*, Table 5.21, Distribution of the population across remoteness areas—30 June 2001, Catalogue No. 1301.0, Australian Bureau of Statistics, Canberra, ABS data used with permission from the Australian Bureau of Statistics; and Australian Bureau of Statistics 2004, Experimental Estimates and Projections, Aboriginal and Torres Strait Islander Australians 1991 to 2009, Estimated Resident Indigenous Population—30 June 2001, page 3 and Table 11, Estimated Resident Indigenous Population by Remoteness Areas—30 June 2001, Catalogue No. 3238.0, Australian Bureau of Statistics, Canberra, ABS data used with permission from the Australian Bureau of Statistics.

The *Australian Government Department of Health and Ageing* is thanked for permission to reproduce the following press releases: Australian Government Department of Health and Ageing, 22 August 2006, *Herceptin*; and Australian Government Department of Health and Ageing, 6 October 2006, *MRI at Sydney Children's Hospital*.

The *Australian Institute of Health and Welfare* is thanked for permission to reproduce material from the Standing Committee on Aboriginal and Torres Strait Islander Health and Statistical Information Management Committee 2006, *National Summary of the 2003 and 2004 Jurisdictional Reports Against the Aboriginal and Torres Strait Islander Health Performance Indicators*, AIHW catalogue No. IHW 16, Australian Institute of Health and Welfare, Canberra, data used with permission from the Australian Institute of Health and Welfare.

The *Commonwealth of Australia* is thanked for permission to present material from the following sources: Productivity Commission 2005, *Australia's Health Workforce*, data from An overview of the current health workforce, pages 333–68, Research Report, Canberra, copyright of Commonwealth of Australia, reproduced by permission; and extracts from Johnson, E. QC, 1991, *Royal Commission into Aboriginal Deaths in Custody National Report*, Volume 1, Section 1.4—The importance of history, <http://www.austlii.edu.au/au/special/ rsjproject/rsjlibrary/rciadic/national/vol1/1.html>, copyright of Commonwealth of Australia, reproduced by permission.

Pearson Education Australia is thanked for permission to reproduce adapted material from Waters, M. & Crook, R. 1993, *Sociology One: Principles of Sociological Analysis for Australians*, 3rd edn, Longman Cheshire, Melbourne, pages 438–9.

Reporters Without Borders is thanked for their permission to reproduce an abbreviated version of the World Press Freedom Index 2006, <http://www.rsf. org>.

Every effort has been made to trace the original source of all material reproduced in this book. Where the attempt has been unsuccessful, the authors and publisher would be pleased to hear from the copyright holder concerned to rectify any omission.

Chapter 1

What is Sociology and Why is it Relevant to Nurses?

Introduction

Julia had always wanted to be a nurse. Her mother and her aunt were both nurses—they had trained in the days when young women lived at 'nurses homes', and they had lots of fun and exciting stories to tell about their training, their time on the wards, and the patients they had looked after. Shift work meant that Julia's mum was home during the day to look after Julia and her two brothers when they were young. But things are different now. Nursing is now taught at university and Julia is the first in her family to study there. Julia doesn't mind too much but her mum is worried that she won't get enough practice on the wards while she trains. Two weeks into the course Julia is starting to worry too—she can understand why she must learn about anatomy and physiology, but she can't see the point of some other subjects. In particular, sociology seems to be completely the wrong subject for nursing. Julia just wants to care for sick people, why should she be thinking about patterns of health and illness, and issues that won't change how she looks after the patients in her care?

A sociological approach to health care shifts the focus from sick individuals to wider social issues; therefore an understanding of sociology enables health care workers to:

- critically evaluate the differing ways that the social world may shape the experience of health and illness
- understand the broader social forces that affect individuals
- consider how health care arrangements impact on the individual's experience of health and illness.

We argue that a sociological understanding of health and illness will result in a more informed approach to the process of health care. Health work occurs in a complex and changing environment. Such changes can be partly attributed to patterns of disease, where long-term chronic illnesses predominate, and partly to variation in the illness experience of different groups in the population. Technological changes mean that hospitalisation may no longer be required for many procedures and, on the other hand, we are able to expand the number of interventions that are possible. Additionally, nurses are working in an environment where the type and cost of care are continually debated in health care organisations and in the public arena. Thus, Julia will need a broad knowledge of health, health care and the organisation of health care if she is to be an effective nurse.

Objectives

After reading this chapter, you should be able to:

- identify the key characteristics of a sociological approach to health issues
- understand why it is important to consider a sociological approach
- have a basic understanding of the differing theoretical perspectives in sociology
- understand some of the key concepts that we will be drawing on in our sociological approach throughout this book.

What is sociology?

Sociology is the study of society. Sociologists identify patterns of behaviour, meanings and beliefs in order to uncover the links between individual lives and social forces, thus revealing how such phenomena are the result of social arrangements at any one time. Importantly, sociology is concerned with the unequal distribution of power and seeks to uncover the effects of this on social life. Understanding social ideas, social structures and power relations enables exploration of how social life is not fixed and unchanging, but was different in the past, varies in different cultures and social settings, and will be different in the future. Williamson (1999: 269) claims that sociology is a reflective discipline that helps to interpret everyday experience and it assists to 'develop nurses who are capable of understanding, analysing and adapting to the social and organizational change which is a chronic feature of our professional lives'.

Approaching sociology: the sociological imagination

The work of C. Wright Mills (1959) points to the need to develop a 'sociological imagination' in order to analyse contemporary social issues. Mills claimed that the sociological imagination enables us to make links between what may seem to be individual issues and their connection with occurrences in society. Using the sociological imagination requires the capacity to look beyond our personal beliefs and experiences, and examine the ways that our personal perspective may be shaped by broader social forces. Thus the sociological imagination '... enables us to grasp history and biography and the relations between the two within society' (Mills, 1959: 6). The sociological imagination provides us with a way of thinking about health and illness issues by considering questions about the relationship of these issues to broader societal forces. This is important when we consider that much of health care provision, and many of the ideas we find in the broader society, focus attention on individuals with problems, rather than locating individuals in a social context that may also contribute to understanding, and solving, health care issues. Pivotal to developing a sociological imagination is the capacity to see the distinction between private troubles and public issues: what may appear to be private troubles, affecting only a few individuals, may in fact be public issues that are of concern to the wider society. While Mills used the example of unemployment to explain the difference, health is replete with examples that can help us to grasp the essence of a sociological imagination.

Consider, for example, the issue of eating disorders in young women (predominantly anorexia nervosa). When viewed as a private trouble, we focus our attention to the individual. Our primary question is: what is it about this young woman's personal psychological state that causes her to starve herself? The solution would be individually focused, as the problem is located in the individual. Therefore, solutions may be sought from the field of nutrition and from psychiatry. However, the statistics on eating disorders indicate that this affliction affects a large number of individuals at any one time in Western cultures, suggesting that this may be a public issue. When anorexia nervosa is seen as a public issue, the question becomes: why is it at this particular time in history and in our culture that young women are choosing to starve themselves? When we turn our attention from the individual to the broader social forces, we identify contributing factors such as gender and body image, the media, and industries that promote particular body shapes and sizes. While we still need to treat individuals who require care, our solutions, even at the individual level, would be better informed because we are locating the illness as a public issue, rather than seeing it as purely individual and psychological.

A sociological perspective requires us to consider the nature of the relationship between individuals and the broader society. In particular, sociologists are interested in the extent to which individuals influence society and society influences individuals. Our social structure develops from the patterns in society that endure over time (such as social class, gender, culture and age) and is an important determinant of life-chances. Social structure can constrain the behaviour of individuals—for example, people from the working class are unlikely to become the prime minister, and women, on average, earn less than men. These examples can be explained in terms of the constraining effects of social class and gender respectively. On the other hand, individuals are able to interpret and give meaning to their social situation in a way that challenges existing social arrangements or creates new ones. This is known as 'agency'. It is important to take account of the constraining effects of social structure as well as the voluntary nature of agency in order to examine social phenomena fully. Encapsulated within sociology as the 'structure–agency' debate, this represents a key challenge in thinking sociologically.

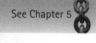
See Chapter 5

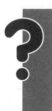

Question for reflection

Identify two health problems that are focused on individuals and their behaviour. How might we see them differently if we viewed these issues as a public issue, rather than as a private trouble?

Sociology and social theory

We can extend our understanding of the sociological approach by considering the importance that sociologists place on social theory in understanding health and illness issues. A theory is a set of ideas that can help to advance knowledge. A theoretical understanding enables us to explain what is happening now and to predict what may happen in the future. Thus, theories in any discipline provide a lens through which we understand the issues at hand. Theories are not static—they are developed and refined through the accumulation of additional knowledge, often through research studies that attempt to apply the theory in a 'real world' setting. We argue that a theoretical knowledge of sociology is useful in health practice settings. Our focus in this book, rather than engaging in debates about the value of one theory over another, is to bridge the gap between theory and practice by illustrating health issues using a range of social theories.

The following description of the recent history of sociology demonstrates the diversity of theories that have been used to understand social issues, particularly as they relate to health and illness, the organisation of health and medical care, and understanding the effects of power differences.

The links between society and health

The differing approaches to health and illness issues can be seen in some of the earliest sociological research and writings. In 1897, French sociologist Emile Durkheim (1858–1917) conducted a study of suicide. While it may be assumed that suicide is an intensely individual act, Durkheim argued that suicide can be understood better by understanding it socially. He found important predictive factors relating to how strongly individuals are integrated into their own society—findings that resonate with contemporary ideas about suicide. From these ideas, a branch of sociology developed theory focusing on how social order and consensus were integral to the smooth functioning of society. Called functionalism, this theoretical approach looked at the broad structures of society to develop ideas about social functioning.

At about the same time, and informed by changes in society brought about by the Industrial Revolution, Karl Marx (1818–83) and Frederick Engels (1820–95) developed a different approach to understanding society. They viewed society as characterised by conflict, not consensus. Engels (1845) charted the poor health conditions of the working classes that had moved into the large cities to work in factories and who suffered from the effects of poor sanitation and overcrowding, combined with unhealthy and unsafe working conditions. Both Marx and Engels focused attention on the ways that society is fundamentally unequal and on how this inequality is evident in patterns of health and illness. The work of Marx and subsequent theorists was further developed in explorations of inequalities in health and illness, and this remains an integral focus in health sociology. Writers from this perspective argue that better health outcomes can only be achieved when the material conditions of disadvantaged groups are improved.

By exploring the links between profit and health care, conflict theorists argue that those in power have little interest in changing social relations to improve health for all. While the focus for many of these theorists is on inequality due to social class, feminist writers have drawn attention to gender inequality. The institution of medicine was also seen as an important contributor to an unequal society. Feminists exposed and critiqued the way that medicine plays an important 'social control' function, thus contributing to the perpetuation of inequalities between men and women.

The work of Max Weber (1864–1920) developed the ideas of Marx by broadening our understanding of inequality. He argued that inequality was not just about economics, but about beliefs, ideals and values. Weber pointed to the importance of understanding 'life chances', an integral component of which is status. He also pointed to the importance of group membership (called 'party'). Thus Weber argued that we needed to understand social inequality by focusing on class, status and party.

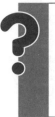

See Chapter 5

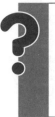

Questions for reflection

Which groups in society do you think are more susceptible to illness? How can we use the theoretical approaches outlined above to begin to explain this?

Sociology in medicine and sociology of medicine

The functionalist view mentioned above was extended by the work of Talcott Parsons (1902–79), a sociologist from the USA. Functionalist research focused on the way in which clearly defined social roles and responsibilities contributed to a structured inequality in society that also serves to maintain consensus. This started a theoretical understanding of the ways in which professions in society have particular roles and status.

See Part 4

One of the most important (and most critiqued) contributions that Parsons made in terms of health was in the development of the 'sick role'. This view sees sickness as 'deviance', in that when people are sick, they are unable to undertake their normal responsibilities. Using the sick role as an explanatory theory helps to explain the mechanisms by which societies are able to allow such deviance. It explains the conditions in society that govern when and under what circumstances we are legitimately allowed to withdraw from normal, social functioning. The sick role theory points to the roles and responsibilities of both patients and professionals in order to minimise the disruptive effects of illness on the smooth functioning of society. Ideas around the 'sick role' theory have resulted in a proliferation of sociological work on issues such as chronic illness, occupational health issues, patient behaviour (including non-compliance) and professions in health.

Writers in the USA continued their focus on sociology in medicine, with particular exploration of professions and professional roles. Renee Fox (1957) developed our theoretical understanding of medical and health knowledge by exploring the concept of 'medical uncertainty'. Other theorists have explored the apparent contradiction between the certainty promised by scientific knowledge and the uncertainty that is experienced in the day-to-day work of doctors and nurses. No two cases will be the same, which raises the question about how we can best educate health care workers for the uncertainties they will face, while at the same time, use a scientific model based on certainty as the cornerstone of their training.

Sociologists have also taken a critical approach to examining the processes by which medicine and medical knowledge have become the dominant form of healing in society today. For example, Elliot Friedson (1970) argued that medicine's position of power in health care was established prior to its use of scientific medicine. In Australia, Evan Willis' (1989) analysis of health care and health care organisations, termed 'medical dominance', examined the ways medicine achieved authority in health care, and other occupations were marginalised as part of this process. This critical exploration of the power of professions in health will be the focus of Part 4 of this book.

 See Part 4

Weber also contributed to sociological theory through his work on professions. He was interested in the ways that different occupations are able to influence the work of others and claim occupational territory of their own. Importantly for our understanding of the contemporary health care organisations that Julia will be working in, Weber (1964) developed our understanding of bureaucracy. While, on the one hand, we need to have rules and procedures in large organisations, Weber also argued that this approach could become an 'iron cage', thus stifling individual creativity in solving problems.

Questions for reflection

Think about your own encounters with health care professionals. What are the defining features of these encounters? Do they vary according to the health care setting?

The experience of illness

Sociological theory has also contributed to our understanding of how individuals understand and experience illness by examining social interaction as it takes place between two or more people. In contrast to structural theories that take a macroperspective by viewing 'society as a whole' and the influence of broad social forces, symbolic interactionism takes a microperspective by focusing attention on the construction of meaning through interaction with others. This approach argues that individuals interpret the world around them, rather than the world being fixed and/or predetermined; that our sense of self (or identity) is produced through interaction with others; and that, through using language or other symbols, we attach meaning to the actions of others. For example, Becker (1963) argued that deviance is a culturally and historically specific condition that depends on certain behaviours being labelled as deviant—thus a deviant act only exists because it is defined as such. In the case of health and illness, a symbolic interactionist approach examines how we interact within the health care system, how we come to define certain conditions as illness, and how these meanings shape our response to specific illnesses. Symbolic interactionism has been important in informing ideas about mental illness because this approach 'focuses on the importance of *power* relations in the *construction* and management of health and illness' (Bilton et al., 1996: 417–18).

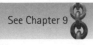
See Chapter 9

The work of Erving Goffman is also important in understanding the experience of illness in contemporary societies. His work on stigma identifies the processes through which some individuals, groups or particular illnesses may be stigmatised (Goffman, 1963). For Goffman, stigma results in a 'spoiled identity'. His work is usefully applied to enhance our understanding of the experience of mental illness, disability and sexually transmitted infections. Similarly, the concept of 'labelling', where one's behaviour is seen in terms of a medical or deviant label, rather than individual attributes, also assists in understanding the experience of, and response to, health and illness issues. Goffman also pointed to the way in which much health and nursing care is comprised of rituals and performances. Important in understanding the experience of being nursed is his idea of 'front stage' and 'back stage' performance. Front stage performances are those situations where people know they are on show and thus they may present themselves in particular socially acceptable ways. However, much nursing work also comprises 'back stage' work where nurses have to assist people with bodily functions and it is difficult, if not impossible, to present these in a socially acceptable manner.

Sociological work on chronic illness has also used the symbolic interaction approach. This work has enabled us to deepen our understanding of how a diagnosis of chronic illness affects our sense of self and thus, the decisions, values and attitudes that may shape our response to such an event. In focusing attention on how we interpret events within a broader social context, sociologists have used symbolic interactionism to explain the effect of chronic illness on identity construction, arguing that we construct our sense of self (our identity) in conjunction with life events, social ideas and values, and interactions with others in society.

 See Chapter 9

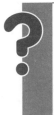

Questions for reflection

Identify contemporary health and/or risk behaviours that may be deemed deviant in our society. Have they always been viewed as deviant? How have ideas about these behaviours changed over time?

Understanding health, understanding knowledge

A number of theories originating in the sociology of knowledge seek to explain how knowledge construction is important in understanding contemporary health care issues. In addition to the ideas about the distribution and experience of illness, some theorists have examined how knowledge shapes our approaches to health and illness. They take as their starting point the idea that our knowledge is contingent upon the social, cultural and historical conditions that exist at any one time. Their theories are therefore focused on 'how we know what we know'. Taking the idea that reality is the product of social, cultural and political interactions, rather than existing independently of them, these theories therefore see medical knowledge and practice as the result of social relations, rather than existing independently in a neutral, objective and value-free scientific vacuum. One of these theories is social construction.

Developed by Berger and Luckmann (1971), the central tenet of social construction is that our knowledge and, in turn, our interpretation of meaning is a result of our social interactions with each other and our environment. This way of viewing the world is useful for critically analysing both our social meanings and the social structure that we may otherwise take for granted. While taking the stance that reality is socially constructed, this approach acknowledges that many illnesses and diseases are biological realities that do exist. As Lupton (2003: 14) points out, the social construction approach 'emphasizes that such experiences are always inevitably given meaning and therefore understood and experienced through cultural and social processes'. Often by highlighting contentious issues, the social construction approach to health and illness points out that health knowledge and power are not objective and value free, but are in fact the result of social ideas and values. For example, there are some areas of life where there are high levels of medical intervention, but where the scientific knowledge informing such intervention is contentious. Examples include attention deficit hyperactivity disorder, menopause and even high blood pressure. Social constructionists are therefore critical of the way in which much of contemporary life has been 'medicalised'—that is, taking areas of our life that were previously not considered as sickness, and applying a medical label and a consequent intervention (often in the form of pharmaceutical drugs).

See Chapters 2 and 10
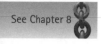

An extension of social construction can be seen in those theories that are 'post-structuralist'. Post-structuralist theories have continued the focus on critically examining health and medical knowledge. The work of the French thinker Michel Foucault (1926–84) has been particularly important in shaping our theories about health knowledge. By taking an historical approach, his work explores the ways that hospitals, clinics and doctors emerged as the key providers of health care. His work also informs contemporary debates in public health about the application of 'lifestyle' knowledge that requires us constantly to focus inwardly on our bodies in order to maintain our health.

See Chapter 8

Importantly, it is through Foucault's development of the idea of 'discourse' that we are able to think about knowledge and ideas in health as being interwoven with health care practice in a way that previous theorists did not. A discourse is a way in which we are able to speak, think and act about an issue. Some discourses are dominant—that is, they are the way we most often approach an issue. For example, a contemporary dominant discourse about cardiac disease is that it relates to lifestyle factors. When we consider the broader patterns of health and illness, we may conclude that heart disease is more about social class than simply lifestyle, but lifestyle is privileged in the way we currently think about heart disease.

Concepts such as medicalisation and discourse alert us to further concepts such as 'ideology' and 'power' that are important in understanding contemporary health and health care issues. The more 'normal' or 'natural' approaches to health problems and their solutions appear to be, the more likely it is that there is general acceptance of these approaches and less inclination to critically examine or question them. A social construction approach would ask questions such as, 'who has constructed this particular knowledge?', 'who stands to benefit from seeing the issue in this way?', and 'how might we think about this differently?'.

In summary, there are different theories in sociology, all of which can assist in explaining aspects of why people do what they do. Some theories are concerned with how social order is maintained in society (e.g. functionalism). Other theories focus on the extent to which access to power means that different groups are advantaged (e.g. conflict theories). Some theories focus on particular aspects of the social structure to try and explore how one's social location can affect life (e.g. feminist theories are concerned with the effect of gender). All of these theories focus their attention on the broader social factors that may affect people's lives.

Other theories in sociology help us to make sense of individual action, meaning and ideas (e.g. symbolic interactionism). Social construction approaches can be seen as a bridge between the broader 'macro-theories' of functionalism and conflict theories, and the 'micro-theories' of symbolic interactionism. By placing knowledge at the centre of this theoretical approach, we can explore both the broader social implications of an issue as well as the experience at the individual level.

Question for reflection

How can an understanding of the social theories outlined above assist Julia (and her classmates) in exploring contemporary health issues?

Our theoretical approach: social construction and critical analysis

While we will point out the contribution of the differing theoretical perspectives throughout the book, theories of social construction inform our approach. We argue that it is important for nurses to develop a critical awareness of the ways in which individuals are shaped by their social world, while at the same time shaping it through their actions. A critical social constructionist approach identifies the ways in which we can bridge the differences between theories that locate explanations in social structure and theories that focus on the individual. To fully understand the links between social structure and individual action we must also examine and analyse the impact of ideas about truth and power.

We argue that we can best analyse contemporary health issues by taking a 'critical approach'. This does not mean that we are using critical in the 'taken-for-granted' sense of criticising everything to do with health. Rather, being critical is about asking why, reflecting on our own social position and questioning the evidence with which we are presented. In trying to see things differently, we may also open up possibilities for change. We agree with Petersen (1994: 5) that when using a critical perspective 'the focus is on power relations between groups and between individuals and on the inequalities that arise from the exercise of power. It draws attention to the power of knowledge to define others and control them, and spells out what this means for health'.

Social constructionism requires that we take a critical perspective in order to consider the power relations that operate around health and illness. How we respond to variations in health status may depend on whether the differential experience is perceived as unfair or inequitable. 'Health inequity refers to those inequalities in health that are deemed to be unfair or stemming from some form of injustice' (Kawachi et al., 2002: 647). Thus, 'health equity is about enabling people to have equitable access to services on the basis of need, it also is about the resources, capacities and power they need to act upon the circumstances of their lives that determine their health' (Keleher & Murphy, 2004: 5).

Question for reflection

Choose a contemporary health issue. What are the key questions you need to ask in taking a 'critical approach' to developing your understanding of the issue?

Using our framework to present a sociological approach for nursing students

This book is in four parts. Part 1 commences our sociological exploration of health and illness by examining ideas about health and illness. Using theory and evidence to understand health and illness, we move beyond a common sense approach or 'taken-for-granted ideas' and question where these ideas come from and who they benefit. For student nurses, this may require a shift in the way they have previously viewed illness issues and the type of health care in contemporary Australia. We start this process by examining what is, in fact, a recent historical approach to health care provision, that of biomedicine. This approach is so dominant that it may be difficult to question or consider alternative viewpoints. One important effect of the discourse of biomedicine is that we tend to locate illness as existing purely within individual motives and action. Sociologists have critiqued the way that this may result in seeing individuals as responsible for their own illnesses, or victim blaming, rather than locating illness issues in the context of broader social structures.

We then shift the focus to exploring other discourses about health that have always existed but that receive less attention than biomedicine. Lay and folk ideas about health can provide health care workers with important information about the people who are in their care. The way that ideas about health and illness are conveyed through the media is examined in the final chapter in Part 1.

In Part 2, we examine the social patterning of health and illness. A sociological approach considers the way that a person's social positioning may affect their life, and in particular, their health. Social structures relate to our position as members of a particular gender, social class, ethnic or indigenous group. Recognising health and illness as socially patterned requires us to question the common-sense idea that illness is the result of 'fate' or simply 'bad luck'. A sociological analysis focuses attention on 'life chances' and the ways that people's health are affected through their membership of particular social groups. We consider the health experiences of a range of population groups by focusing on the issues of social marginalisation and exclusion. Sensitised to the issues of social patterning and to freedom of choice (the structure–agency debate), Julia should be able to weigh up just how much social circumstances can impact on issues of access, equity and equality in health care.

Part 3 focuses on the experience of illness. We start by questioning what it means to be healthy or ill, and, using the sociology of the body, examine how concepts such as 'risk' and 'lifestyle' and ideas about the 'normal healthy body' shape our understandings of health and illness. An important change in health care patterns is the increase in chronic illness. The onset, diagnosis and treatment of chronic illnesses are as much social experiences as medical phenomena. A sociological perspective incorporates both individual and social responses to chronic illnesses. Such a perspective is useful for health workers to understand the links between people's perceptions and their decisions in the face of chronic illness. Further, our experience of health care is likely to be shaped by prevailing trends in technological development. We explore the issues associated with the increased technological intervention in the definition, diagnosis and treatment of illness through case studies of genetics and pharmaceuticals.

Finally, in Part 4 we examine the complex array of organisations that make up contemporary health care. Any attempt to explore current health issues must take account of health care as a social institution. The provision of health care is also 'big business' and contemporary health care is expensive. The way that a society organises health care provision is indicative of the values that society holds about social and individual responsibility, prevention versus cure and, most importantly, the extent to which business interests are able to exert power over the constitution of disease and medical interventions. These issues are particularly important for nurses as they become key players in the provision of health care through moves towards professionalisation, as evidenced in tertiary education and in the changing roles of nurses.

CONCLUSION

Sociology offers an alternative theoretical lens, one that is reflective, critical and questioning, in order to reveal social factors influencing the causes, experiences and consequences of contemporary health and illness patterns. This is important for nurses working in a world of social change, and understanding about illness, not just task-based learning, is seen as a vital part of being a nurse in contemporary society. Nursing is more than the technical skill that Julia's mother is envisioning, for which the key component in learning is to practice. Nursing curricula require that students get sufficient practice in caring for people in hospital wards and community-based settings, but because nursing courses are educating nurses for entry to a profession, they also require students to be critical and reflective in their understanding of the ideas about health and illnesses, the social forces that predispose population groups to particular risks and illnesses, and the wider context of the health system in which they will work. Thus, we concur with Porter (1997: 217) that 'sociological knowledge should be an intrinsic component of nursing knowledge ... [because] nursing involves the social interaction of human individuals'.

REVIEW QUESTIONS

1   How does applying the sociological imagination change the way in which you view contemporary health issues?
2   Choose one of the social theories listed in this chapter. How does it contribute to your understanding of health and illness?
3   What is meant when we argue that health and illness are 'socially constructed'? Use an example to illustrate your answer.

KEY TERMS

1 Theories

Conflict theory
Feminist
Functionalism
Post-structuralism
Social construction
Symbolic interaction

2 Concepts

Bureaucracy
Deviance
Discourse
Gender
Ideology
Inequality

Labelling
Life chances
Medicalisation
Medical dominance
Medical uncertainty
Power
Professions
Public issues and private troubles
Sick role
Social structure and agency
Sociological imagination
Social class
Stigma
Victim blaming

FURTHER READING

1 Introductory texts on sociology

Van Krieken, R., Habibis, D., Smith, P., Hutchins, B., Haralambos, M. and Holborn, M. 2006, *Sociology: Themes and Perspectives*, Frenchs Forest, Pearson Education Australia.

Willis, E. 2004, *The Sociological Quest: An Introduction to the Study of Social Life*, Crows Nest, Allen & Unwin.

2 Texts on the sociology of health and illness

Barry, A.M. and Yuill, C. 2002, *Understanding Health: A Sociological Introduction*, London, Sage.

Cheek, J., Shoebridge, J., Willis, E. and Zadoroznyj, M. 1996, *Society and Health: Social Theory for Health Workers*, Longman, Melbourne.

Germov, J. (ed.) 2005, *Second Opinion: An Introduction to Health Sociology*, South Melbourne, Oxford University Press.

Gray, D.E. 2006, *Health Sociology: An Australian Perspective*, Frenchs Forest, Pearson Education.

Grbich, C. (ed.) 2004, *Health in Australia: Sociological Concepts and Issues*, Frenchs Forest, Pearson Education.

Keleher, H. and Murphy, B. (eds) 2004, *Understanding Health: A Determinants Approach*, South Melbourne, Oxford University Press.

Lupton, D. 2003, *Medicine as Culture*, Sage, London.

Nettleton, S. 1995, *The Sociology of Health & Illness*, Cambridge, Polity Press.

Petersen, A.R. 1994, *In a Critical Condition: Health and Power Relations in Australia*, St Leonards, Allen & Unwin.

Part 1

Ideas about Health and Illness

In Part 1 of this book we draw attention to the social practices, processes, values and beliefs that inform ideas about health and illness. By examining the basis for our explanatory frameworks, we highlight the many different ways in which health and illness can be conceptualised. This part looks at the diversity of ideas that inform health and health actions, first by contrasting a sociological and biomedical approach, then by exploring lay perceptions of health (including cross-cultural and indigenous health beliefs), and finally by examining how the media constructs ideas and meanings about health and illness.

The first chapter in this part, 'Approaching Health and Illness', provides a critical analysis of the dominant scientific ideas that contribute to our understanding of health and illness. In this way we expose the socially constructed nature of health and illness, and the ways that our approaches to health and illness are shaped by social, historical and political factors. We extend our discussion of the socially constructed nature of health and illness in Chapter 3, 'Lay, Folk and Consumer Ideas about Health and Illness', which illustrates the influence of culture on ideas about health and healing. This chapter concludes with a discussion about the way that health care consumers' knowledge has increased, thereby changing their expectations of health care. The final chapter in this part, 'The Media and Health', examines the role of the media as a source of knowledge for health care consumers. We also demonstrate how the media influences our own understanding of health and illness as well as shapes the health and illness experience of others.

Chapter 2

Approaching Health and Illness

Introduction

Health knowledge is often viewed as scientific knowledge. The dominance of science as the guiding discipline for medical ideas means that it is often difficult to look past what are presented as facts and to explore alternative knowledge sources or the social factors that may contribute to the medical worldview. A sociological approach to health and medical knowledge critically evaluates the basis of such an understanding. This is known as the sociology of knowledge approach and it enables an examination of what we know as 'truth' and explores whether the facts that we believe in so strongly may be more the result of social, cultural and historical processes, than an infallible and authoritative view of the world.

In this chapter, we take a critical look at the framework that is most commonly drawn upon in our understanding of health and illness. In order to do so, we begin by reflecting on the idea of 'truth' and introduce the idea of discourse as a useful way of examining health and illness ideas. We then examine the set of ideas that comprises what is known as 'biomedicine'. Subjecting the ideas that inform biomedicine to further examination comprises the sociological critique of biomedicine. This critique has emerged as ideas about biomedicine have been contested. Finally, we examine the key points that a sociological analysis of health and illness can bring to our understanding of health and health care issues. Sociological theories can help us to identify the socially constructed nature of health and illness, and the ways that our approaches to health and illness are shaped by social, historical and political factors.

Objectives

After reading this chapter, you should be able to:

■ discuss the difference between a biomedical and sociological approach to health and illness
■ critically analyse the dominant ideas that contribute to our understanding of health and illness
■ apply your understanding of the different ideas about health and illness to contemporary health issues.

Key ideas: knowledge, discourse, power and truth

A defining characteristic of sociology is its critical and questioning approach to understanding our social world. As part of our social world, health care and medicine are comprised of ideas, theories and practices that change over time, reflecting changing social ideas, values and priorities. Health and medical explanations may also vary across differing cultures. It is these historical, social and cultural dimensions of health and medical knowledge that lead us to question how knowledge of health issues is constructed, the processes of acceptance or 'legitimacy' that accrue to particular explanations, and the consequences of the dominance of such explanations.

One way of understanding the many ideas that shape what we know is to use the concept of 'discourse'. A discourse 'represents a distinct way of thinking, seeing and conversing about a particular phenomena, all of which create a virtual "arena"' (Barry & Yuill, 2002: 15). A discourse is more than language—it comprises the ideas that contribute to making meaning about a topic, the ways in which we speak about it, as well as the types of action that are enabled by such thoughts and language. At any particular time, certain discourses will be dominant. These are the ideas and practices that carry more weight or legitimacy and they can be described as 'dominant discourses'. These are the ideas that are most socially accepted as the 'right' way to think about issues, categories of people, social factors and behaviour.

The power of discourse lies in the authority and power that can be exercised when one's ideas, values and explanations are accepted as the 'right' way of understanding an issue. At a practical level in health care, resources flow to those who are able to convince us of the 'rightness' of their approach. Dominant discourses have legitimacy in the explanations they provide. At any one time, there may be multiple discourses about an issue, thus a dominant discourse may change as competing explanations achieve legitimacy. When we think about knowledge as discourses, we start to explore how there may be many competing ways of understanding an issue. As we see in this chapter and the next, there are many different discourses about health and illness, and they vary in their degrees of influence and authority.

See Chapter 3

Sociological enquiry seeks to understand how some discourses achieve legitimacy and become dominant. The use of discourse in the analysis of health care is attributed to a key social theorist, Foucault, who was interested in the relationship between knowledge and power and how this shapes social reality. Foucault's analysis of knowledge and power provides an understanding of how knowledge and discourses both operate to legitimise power. In other words, 'claims to knowledge and authority by proponents of certain discourses are thus in effect claims to power' (Cheek et al., 1996: 174). The knowledge and power vested in particular discourses serves to limit or exclude alternative discourses. Petersen (1994) argues that the sociology of health is about health and power relations, and knowledge enables 'power over others' (Petersen, 1994: 6).

This means that we should look at the idea of 'truth' and knowledge in a critical way. The idea of discourse, and the fact that there may be competing discourses, helps us to unravel the idea that there may be many competing claims to 'truth' and that the idea of obtaining legitimacy for one's truth is an exercise in power. Thus, in critiquing the idea of truth, it is argued that: 'What is asserted to be "truth" should be considered the product of power relations, and as such, is never neutral, but always acting in the interests of someone' (Lupton, 2003: 12). It is through this approach to critically analysing 'what counts' as knowledge that we approach dominant ideas about health and illness. In order to do this we will first examine the rise of scientific medicine in Western societies.

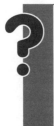

Questions for reflection

Consider the way that pregnancy and childbirth have invoked the use of medical technologies (e.g. ultrasound, genetic testing, epidural, caesarean, foetal monitoring). What are the dominant discourses about pregnancy and childbirth? How do these discourses legitimise the use of technology? What competing discourses have been marginalised?

The discourses of science and scientific medicine

The discourses of science and scientific medicine are very influential and are considered authoritative in most Western societies. In examining the historical development of the scientific discourse and its influence on the development of modern medicine, it will become evident that the scientific knowledge that underpins modern medicine is a product of its history and social context.

The causes of health and illness have long been linked to the supernatural and nature. Supernatural causes of health and illness had (and arguably still have) a very strong influence and led to the development of beliefs, superstitions and religious rituals. These may include, for example, gazing into a crystal ball to discover the intentions of the supernatural in order to cast a magic spell, or to induce vomiting or other forms of cure. Not everyone was gifted with the special abilities to diagnose or cure illnesses in this way, and those which could obtained positions of power because of their ability to intercede with the supernatural. These people were known variously as shamans, witch doctors or medicine men. Some of these healers became very knowledgeable and learned in their craft. Thus, religion, cultural practices and medicine became inextricably linked and this had significant implications for both those who practised medicine (seen as akin to the gods) and those who became sick (seen as sinners or possessed by evil).

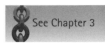 See Chapter 3

4
Humours.

 Natural (biological) causes of illness and disease were advocated by Hippocrates (460–377 BC) and he is credited with being 'the father of medicine'. Hippocrates located the cause of disease within the body and claimed that the role of the physician was to assist the body to heal by helping the body restore its natural balance. This was a significant shift from viewing physicians as having 'special powers' to physicians as aiding the body's natural recovery; and from sinners to sick people. Hippocrates also called for a more compassionate and ethical approach to medicine. This is illustrated in the Hippocratic Oath. The central tenet of this oath—do no harm—while not always pledged by modern doctors, persists within modern medicine. Another important figure in ancient medicine was 'the Father of Experimental Physiology', Galen (129–200 AD), a Roman physician who contributed to knowledge about anatomy by dissecting monkeys and pigs (the use of human cadavers was illegal), and proved many commonly held ideas about human anatomy to be wrong.

It was not until the Enlightenment period in the eighteenth century that superstitious and religious beliefs about the causes of illness were challenged. During the Enlightenment, there was a body of thought that was committed to applying reason to human life in order to develop rational, secular and scientific explanations. Also referred to as the scientific revolution, this era saw scientific methods of observation and experimentation applied to natural life to produce unbiased, objective and rational evidence. Karl Popper (1902–94), a philosopher of science, argued that a theory is truly scientific if it is observable, measurable, refutable,[1] repeatable and predictable. Thus, the study of the human body and disease causation became truly scientific. The zealous pursuit of scientific knowledge resulted in rapid advancements, even though the resultant changes in practice were much slower.

Further development of modern medicine was influenced by the settings in which medical care took place. The rapid increase in the number of hospitals in the 1800s gave rise to increased opportunities to observe patients clinically. The application of the scientific method in medicine led to a greater use of the

---

1   The aim should be to disprove rather than prove since verification is impossible because of the infinite number of variables that may affect the test.

laboratory for observation and experimentation. The discovery of the cell by Rudolf Virchow (1821–1902) unlocked important clues for the links between anatomy, physiology and pathology. Also in the laboratory, Louis Pasteur (1822–95) discovered that bacteria are not spontaneously generated, and this spurred other bacteriological discoveries. Other advancements were made in the operating theatre, which provided ample opportunity to observe and learn from the functioning of live bodies. This led to developments in the area of anaesthesia, pain control, infection control and the localised nature of disease (Weiss & Lonnquist, 2006).

From the historical development of medicine, it is evident that the focus on understanding disease causation began with a consideration of the whole person and their relationship with their world, and spiralled down to focusing on a cellular level. Along the way, precedence has been given to gaining scientific knowledge through observation and experimentation. The increasingly scientific nature of medicine placed it within the domain of people who had access to education and training, and systematically excluded lay practitioners from its practice. Focusing on the disease or cellular dysfunction also had the effect of portraying disease as a neutral state devoid of any moral, ethical, social, political and historical meanings (White, 1991).

Biomedicine: a dominant discourse

The development of medicine in response to infectious diseases led to the acceptance by the medical profession and the general population that illness and disease are a result of an individual's biology. Medical knowledge and practices based on the supernatural were eventually discarded, or at least scorned, in favour of new scientific knowledge. The historical development of medicine in the Western world has resulted in the dominance of the biomedical model. The discourse of biomedicine features prominently in our health care system. The following discussion outlines the key features of this approach to health and healing.

Doctrine of specific aetiology

In this model, illness or disease is caused by identifiable biological forces. This theory of disease causation has its origins in the positivist Enlightenment period when the agents responsible for diseases, such as cholera, syphilis and typhoid, were discovered. It has become known as the doctrine of specific aetiology. Thus, illness or disease is seen to have a specific cause and treatment should alleviate all symptoms.

The body as a machine

The early attempts at developing an understanding of how the body works led to a focus on discovering how the component parts of the body function. The body was seen as a compilation of interrelated parts and came to be viewed in a mechanistic way, as a machine. As a consequence, illness or disease was viewed as a malfunction and the focus narrowed to considering how to remedy the broken part, rather than the person as a whole. Metaphors portraying the body as a machine continue to prevail—for example, 'lean mean fighting machine'; 'a breakdown'; 'the heart as a pump'; 'body clock'. These mechanical metaphors also reflect the doctor's actions in repairing the body—for example, 'patch it up'; 'put you back together'; 'clean out your pipes'; 'fix your water works'; 'turn back the clock'; 'fix your ticker'.

Mind–body distinction

As a consequence of the focus on the anatomical structures of the body, the physical body is considered separately from the mind. This is referred to as the mind–body distinction or Cartesian dualism. Seventeenth-century philosopher René Descartes (1596–1650) devoted much of his life to trying to prove that the body operates independently from the mind. His work profoundly influenced the development of scientific medicine and embedded the notion that the body can be viewed as a machine without reference to psychological, emotional or spiritual influences. As a result, doctors paid less attention to the psycho-social dimensions of illness.

Reductionist

The biomedical model is, thus, a reductionist model, or in other words, the body is reduced to its component parts. Ahn et al. (2006: 956) explain that reductionism is a useful guiding principle but it 'becomes less effective when the act of dividing a problem into its parts leads to loss of important information about the whole'. The experience of being sick is reduced to a biochemical or anatomical occurrence, and is unrelated to social factors. In this way, illness or disease is something that happens to parts of the body, not the whole person. The pitfalls of the reductionist approach may be less evident in the case of an acute illness or simple disease with an identifiable cause and specific intervention than in the case of chronic or complex diseases. This predominance of focusing on the body's particular parts and body systems is evident in the way that medical specialties have emerged and even the way that hospitals are organised into departments—for example, obstetrics, renal, orthopaedic and cardiac.

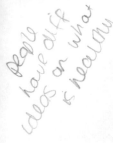

People have diff. ideas on what is healthy.

Narrow definition of health

Within the biomedical model, health is defined as the absence of disease. Disease or illness is viewed as a dysfunction, or a deviation from the normal body. If our body part is functioning within the normal range, then we are considered to be healthy. This also assumes that there is a defined normal range and that 'normal' is readily identifiable.

Individualistic

The biomedical model focuses on the disease and illness of individuals. This is encouraged through its focus on locating the sources of the illness within the individual's body rather than within the broader social environment.

Treatment versus prevention

The biomedical model is a curative model. The preoccupation with diagnosis and intervention means that its primary purpose is treatment or cure rather than prevention. For example, in the case of a person with wrist pain, a doctor may perform surgery or prescribe anti-inflammatory drugs rather than investigate the cause in order to prevent the recurrence of the pain. If the community is given a choice between employing two health promotion nurses or purchasing resuscitation equipment for an ambulance, the chances are that it will choose the ambulance. The likelihood of this occurring is due to discourses that privilege ideas about treatment and cure over those of prevention.

Treatment imperative

The idea that medicine can 'fix the broken part' has led to a strong compulsion to seek medical intervention to regain normal functioning and health. This treatment imperative drives the search for the best intervention or cure, for the 'magic bullet' that will address the specific cause of the disease. These treatments and cures are necessarily the product of science and underpinned by the notion that they are proven and effective.

Neutral scientific process

Guiding principles of the scientific approach emphasise its rationality, value neutrality and objectivity. These principles are evident in the way that medical knowledge is constructed and medicine is practised. Medical knowledge is gained from observation and experimentation. Knowledge is only accepted into the medical community once it has been scientifically proven. The randomised control trial[2] remains the 'gold standard' of evidence within the medical community. The way doctors practise medicine is also meant to be objective and replicable. In this way, different doctors with the same medical training and education who apply the same diagnostic tools should reach the same conclusion about a patient's illness. There is an assumption that these processes are devoid of any subjective (or personal) judgments.

While each of these characteristics can be seen as quite distinct, they share a disregard for social factors. A sociological perspective allows us to 'debunk' some of the taken-for-granted ideas that shape these discourses and to think about how social factors might be at work in health and illness.

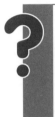

Question for reflection

Make a list of the advantages and disadvantages of a health system where biomedicine is the dominant discourse. Do the advantages outweigh the disadvantages?

A sociological perspective

The biomedical model has been the subject of much critique and debate, and a sociological perspective on health and illness provides an alternative view. Lupton (2003) argues that the relevance of understanding health using sociology has occurred, primarily, for three reasons: first, there has been a disillusionment with the promises of scientific medicine. Challenged by complexity and uncertainty in many contemporary health problems, the biomedical approach has not provided the solutions promised by advances in science and technology. Second, claims that medicine is not always effective, and sometimes not always benevolent, have led to a critique of the use of medicine as a social institution, particularly as an agent of social control. The role of doctors in Nazi Germany exposed the ways that medicine could be co-opted. Finally, the idea that knowledge, even medical knowledge, is not neutral has pointed to the need to understand the power relations that affect health care decision making.

Sociologists point to the effects of biomedicine being the dominant discourse about health. For example, with a focus on specific aetiology, the social aetiology

---

2   'In its simplest form, patients are randomly assigned to a group receiving the treatment under investigation and to a control group receiving standard treatment, a placebo or no treatment at all. If the two groups are initially the same, and then are treated in exactly the same way in all other respects, any difference in outcome must be attributable to the treatment' (Daly, 2005: 5–6).

of disease is largely ignored. This means that the social and political conditions that contribute to ill health receive little attention and, in effect, the domain of health becomes 'depoliticised'. As a result of the primacy given to the biomedical model, little attention is paid (and therefore fewer resources are given) to addressing the broader determinants of health—for example, housing, education, employment and environment.

Defining health as the absence of disease is also flawed in light of the current knowledge that some people may have the specific biological factor that causes disease but do not develop any symptoms. For example, the germs that cause meningococcal disease can be found in the nose and throat of up to 20 per cent of the population but usually these people do not go on to develop the disease. There are also many other ways of defining health other than normal biological functioning. For example, the World Health Organization (1948) defines health as 'a state of complete physical, mental and social well-being and not merely the absence of disease or infirmity'.

The socially constructed nature of medical knowledge

Sociologists also argue that medical knowledge is socially constructed, arguing that medical knowledge is influenced by society and, therefore, is not scientifically neutral. This is evident in the way that medical knowledge and the practice of medicine have changed over time as a result of changing ways of understanding our social world through history or culture.

While the science that informs biomedicine is seen to deal only with the production of 'facts', a sociological perspective points to the way that facts are constructed. Kuhn (1962) coined the term 'paradigm' to refer to a particular frame of reference. He argues that scientific activities occur within a particular scientific paradigm that determines what the problems are, what the solutions are likely to look like and how we should go about looking for the answers. In this way, the subject and process of scientific discovery are shaped according to the values, beliefs, techniques and so on—the paradigm—shared by the particular scientific community.

Over time, scientists gather knowledge within their particular scientific paradigm. Kuhn challenges the notion that scientific knowledge is cumulative; rather he argues that new discoveries that are not consistent with the existing paradigm cause a paradigm shift. He refers to these paradigm shifts as scientific revolutions that represent a break from the earlier accepted theory and require new ways of thinking about the subject and process of scientific study—that is, a new paradigm. Tension occurs when scientists find that the evidence they are gathering does not fit with their existing paradigm but they are reluctant to discard it until a new and better one appears. Kuhn went so far as to suggest that as a result of their value bias, scientists may cling so tightly to their existing theories that it is only when the generation of scientists attached to the old theory have retired that the new theory will replace it.

Kuhn's work helps to explain that the scientific basis of medical knowledge is a collective knowledge of those who subscribe to a particular scientific paradigm. These paradigms determine the type of questions that are asked and the methods that are used. It is not until there is a shift in thinking or a paradigm shift that new ways of understanding are possible. Fleck (1896–1961) pointed out that changes in thinking about the germ theory of disease causation did not occur until there were 'thought collectives' (akin to paradigms) to embrace it, even though it was well known that not everyone who had germs contracted disease (Cheek et al., 1996). More recent application of the concept of paradigms suggests that within the field of medicine, the various medical specialty areas exist within different paradigms and, in a similar way, even within the broad field of health, health professionals operate from different paradigms.

These differing paradigms of knowledge are illustrated in the story of stomach ulcers. Explanations and treatment for ulcers originally focused on psychological causes. From the 1950s, discoveries in biology led to a focus on lifestyle (in particular stress and diet), with those affected advised to control their diet, avoid 'rich' and spicy foods, and minimise other foods that may irritate the stomach. Coexisting with this explanation from the 1970s came drug therapies that were aimed at reducing the production of acid in the stomach, thus eliminating the need for restrictive diets if sufferers persisted in their use of these drugs (these included Tagamet and Zantac), which helped to heal but not cure the ulcers. In 1979, the knowledge about ulcers again changed when it was discovered that ulcers may be bacterial in origin, and thus amenable to short-term antibiotic treatment. This new knowledge was contrary to the previous belief that bacteria could not survive in the stomach's acid environment. However, there was a long time-lag between the discovery of the bacteria *Helicobacter pylori* and changes in the management of stomach ulcers.

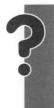

Questions for reflection

Why do you think that the discovery of the bacterial cause of ulcers did not immediately change the most common treatment for this illness? What does this case study tell us about scientific paradigms and new knowledge?

The side effects of a dominant discourse

A sociological perspective on biomedicine as a dominant discourse also points to the harmful effects of such dominance. This can be through the social responsibilities that we delegate to the institution of medicine (social control); side effects, inappropriate or harmful use (iatrogenesis); the expansion of medical explanations into areas of our social life (medicalisation); and the effects of locating causes of health solely within individuals (victim blaming).

Medicine and social control

A sociological perspective of health and illness goes beyond the illness experience of the individual to also explore the social, cultural and political factors that impact on their experience of the health care system. A sociological perspective points to the ways in which diagnosis and treatment are social processes. While medical knowledge is portrayed socially as arising from disinterested and politically neutral sources, its origin and implementation are based very much around social processes and social institutions. One way that we can observe this is in the use of medicine as an institution of social control. Social control is a process by which social stability is maintained through the exercise of sanctions, compliance or commitment to a shared world view. As noted in the introduction, the work of Talcott Parsons is important in illustrating the ways that medicine plays an important social function in controlling access to the 'sick role'. In this regard, illness is seen as a deviation from the normal and the role of medicine is to ensure that only people who are legitimately ill are excused from their normal duties.

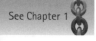

See Chapter 1

However, social control can be effected in other ways. By extending the domain of sickness, people can be excluded from activities on the basis of being unwell. Feminist researchers have pointed to the ways that medicine has effectively acted as a social control agent over women. For example, in the mid 1800s in America, medical theories about women's finite energy reserve and their predisposition to 'hysteria' meant that they were excluded from public social life and unable to vote or engage in higher education. Further, the exclusion of women on medical grounds meant that the malice of oppression was taken out of this form of social control (Ehrenreich & English, 1978). Contemporary examples of the way that medicine acts as an agent of social control include the role of medical expertise in deciding whether people should be deemed eligible for some welfare payments and other supports, legitimating time off work, or even legitimating the incapacity to complete university assignments on time!

Iatrogenesis

Sociologists have also critiqued the way that medicine may actually be harmful for health. Iatrogenesis means illness originating in the healer. In a radical critique of medicine, Ivan Illich (1976) argued that such iatrogenesis can be found at the clinical, social and cultural levels in society. At the clinical level, iatrogenic illness may occur through the use of medical technology and diagnostic testing, the overuse of medical and surgical procedures, and the use of pharmaceutical drugs. The doctrine of specific aetiology suggests we can identify the causative organism, but unfortunately this does not mean that we can isolate the causative organism from the rest of the body; therefore, medical interventions may impact on much more than the affected part. For example, pharmaceutical drugs can have side effects and often people are prescribed other drugs to counter the side effects, which may themselves have side effects. This is known as 'cascade iatrogenesis'. Elderly people are at increased risk because they may have more than one illness (co-morbidities) and their ability to metabolise drugs is diminished. Non-steroidal anti-inflammatory drugs (like ibuprofen, indomethacin) are commonly given for arthritis; however, they may cause stomach ulcers and renal impairment, particularly in elderly people.

Illich (1976) also argued that iatrogenesis occurs at a broader social level, arguing that medicine has actually been detrimental to people's health due to the expansion of medical services in such a way that we are encouraged to become consumers of a 'quick medical fix', and that health issues have been expanded to include a broad range of social problems. The promises of biomedicine mean that pharmaceutical and surgical interventions become the normal approach to illness (and carry with them their own rates of iatrogenesis), rather than looking at the social conditions that create a 'morbid' society. At an even broader level, it is argued that our reliance on medicine means that culturally we struggle to come to terms with the reality of living in our contemporary world, particularly around death and dying, because all events become medical events. Such incapacity to deal with values around pain, death and dying are, Illich argues, harmful to society.

Medicalisation

To suggest that illness and disease are social constructions also suggests that some people have the power to define them as such. Within our society, this power is vested in the medical profession. The dominance of medical ideas and the high level of social acceptance of the biomedical discourse has led to an increasing level of influence of medical ideas in our social lives.

Conrad (1992: 209) defines medicalisation as a 'process by which nonmedical problems become defined and treated as medical problems, usually in terms of illnesses or disorders'. Conrad goes on to argue that the key factors in this process are in the definition of a problem, the use of language to describe it and intervening

case study

Julia went to hospital to visit her cousin Maria, who had just had a baby. Julia was surprised to learn that Maria had given birth by caesarean as she had been planning a natural birth. She asked her cousin about the events that led to the caesarean. Maria explained that as she was about a week overdue, she was brought into the hospital to have her labour induced. This started with the insertion of gel onto her cervix. She had a few 'niggles' but labour didn't really start, so Maria was sent home to rest overnight and see if anything happened. At home Maria was anxious, restless and couldn't sleep. She came back to the hospital in the morning for a check. The midwife examined her and said that her cervix had softened but was only very slightly dilated.

Around lunch time, the contractions were stronger but there was no regular pattern. They suggested starting a drip to bring the labour on. With the drip in her arm, Maria found it difficult to walk around. The contractions also quickly became more forceful and painful. By late afternoon, Maria was starting to get very tired, especially after very little sleep the night before. They were also frequently monitoring the baby, which meant that Maria had to lie still so the monitor could be attached. By dinner time the labour was progressing but slowly and the pain was getting too much for Maria. She finally agreed to an epidural. Maria said it was weird not being able to feel anything but the relief was good. She slept for a little while. She was woken while the monitor was attached again and she was examined. The midwife said the baby was starting to show signs of distress during the contractions. The epidural was turned down so that Maria had more feeling and could push, but the baby still wouldn't come out. They told her it was in 'a bad position'.

Maria finally had her baby delivered by caesarean at just after midnight. Maria told Julia she wondered how it might have been different if she had been able to sleep the night before and if she had been able to move around freely during her labour. She also told Julia that even though she thought she had prepared well for the birth, she had found it very frightening and that because of this fear she found it impossible to ask questions about the interventions that were suggested because she was afraid for the well-being of her baby.

Questions

Does Maria's story illustrate iatrogenesis and/or medicalisation? What are the reasons for your answer?

to treat the problem using a medical framework. This may apply to biological events previously regarded as natural occurrences and not given a disease label, such as pregnancy, childbirth and menopause. For example, menopause is no longer considered a natural life process. It has been redefined as an oestrogen-deficient disease for which there is an increasing number of remedies and treatments that should be used. Medicalisation is also said to apply to those life experiences that have generally been considered in the domain of the social. Increasingly, sociologists have been critical of the ways that medicalisation has been applied to behaviours or social problems, using case studies relating to alcoholism, hyperactivity, mental illness, compulsive gambling and transsexualism. Considered an extreme example, the medicalisation of compulsive buying highlights whether such a medical label is an individual psychological disorder or a symptom of a wider societal problem of consumerism (Lee & Mysyk, 2004).

One way to explore the concept of medicalisation is to focus on the extent to which 'normal healthy' people become subject to a medical diagnosis. Consider a continuum. At one end are people who are suffering from a particular condition, who need a diagnosis and treatment. While we may debate what form of treatment is most appropriate, few would deny that a medical diagnosis offers relief and some intervention. In the middle of the continuum, we may find people with varying signs and symptoms of the same condition that may cause some discomfort but for whom medical diagnosis and intervention may or may not be necessary. At the other end of the continuum is the 'normal healthy population' who have no signs or symptoms of the condition. The issue with medicalisation is often not whether a disease or illness should receive a label and treatment, but the extent to which the range of those deemed in need of medical intervention extends along the continuum to the 'normal healthy' end. The question becomes where does 'normal and healthy' finish and illness start? Current (and controversial) examples of the 'medicalisation along the continuum approach' are menopause, attention deficit (hyperactivity) disorder and anxiety.

Medicalisation is illustrative of the dominance of the discourse of biomedicine. It not only reflects the power and interests of the medical profession, but may also be the result of other interests in health. For example, the designation of a medical label may bring legitimacy for people who are seeking acknowledgment of their suffering. Thus, activists have advocated for chronic fatigue syndrome to be legitimised as an illness. Other influences on the process of medicalisation include the industries that benefit from the legitimacy accorded to an illness. For example, medicalisation rarely occurs in the absence of an intervention to solve the problem, and pharmaceutical companies are influential players in the determination of both the disease and the solution.

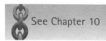
See Chapter 10

Victim blaming

A key contribution of sociology to debates about health and illness lies in the understanding of historical, structural and cultural factors that shape the illness experience. A biomedical focus locates illness in the attributes of an individual—either psychological, genetic or biological. One consequence of this can be 'victim blaming', where individuals are seen as primarily responsible for their ill health. The action that follows from such an explanation focuses on 'changing the victim' rather than bringing about social change. The structuring of medical services as highly individualised in their approach and treatment contributes to seeing illness as an individual attribute. Sociologists argue that individual action (or agency) may be influenced by many factors. In relation to the social distribution of health and illness, it is argued that one's structural position in society (social class, gender, ethnicity and age) greatly influence health, and that individual action and responsibility for health is mediated not only by our position in society, but also the social and cultural responses to illness.

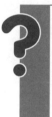

See Chapter 5

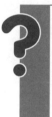

Question for reflection

Return to the list you constructed earlier about the advantages and disadvantages of biomedicine. To what extent do the issues raised by the sociological critique of biomedicine undermine the advantages?

A sociological approach to health and illness

Thus, in addition to questioning the dominant discourses about health and medicine, and critiquing the consequences of over-reliance on biomedicine, the appeal of a sociological approach to health and illness lies in its ability to provide a holistic portrayal of people and their health issues. Whereas the primary concern of the biomedical model is the physical body, the primary concern of a sociological perspective of health and illness is the social. Thus, someone who has diabetes is not just someone with a chronic condition; they may also have a family, a job and a partner, as well as an emotional and spiritual dimension. In this way, a sociological approach seeks to redress some of the criticisms of the reductionist and mechanistic features of the biomedical model.

It is difficult for sociology to challenge the dominant biomedical portrayals of illness and disease because the discourse of scientific knowledge in constructing truth means that medicine is seen as a major source of truth in our society (Petersen, 1994). To use our sociological imagination in this instance is to put aside our belief in scientific medicine and be open to exploring the social processes that are inherent within it. How then is illness defined from a sociological perspective? While not denying individual biology, a social construction perspective focuses on the way that an illness comes to be defined as such, the knowledge that informs such a definition, the interests that may benefit from such a definition and the social patterning of the illness.

case study

Anita and John have two sons, Will aged 7 years and Tom aged 4 years. John is a marketing executive with a multinational food company who works long hours and is often away from home on business trips. Anita works part time as a graphic designer for a local advertising company and her work hours are more flexible than John's. Their home life is very busy as they juggle work and family commitments.

Anita has become increasingly concerned about her eldest son. Will had always been an active little boy but she thought this was normal for boys. However, lately his behaviour has become a problem. His inability to follow directions and stay focused on getting ready for school in the mornings creates havoc when things need to go smoothly so they can all get to work and school on time. Anita spends a large part of her work day feeling guilty for yelling at Will in anger and frustration because he invariably loses part of his school uniform somewhere in transition from the bedroom to the lounge room to the car.

She knows that yelling doesn't do any good; it certainly doesn't seem to change his behaviour and it upsets Tom as well. Tom asked Anita to go to the shopping centre the other day for a milkshake and a hot dog, complaining that it had been ages since they had been there. Anita thought about this and realised that he was right, it had been a long time. Will's behaviour in public was nightmarish and she had actively avoided going to crowded places with him. The last time they went to the shopping centre, while Anita was getting some money from the ATM, Will put Tom in a supermarket trolley and was about to release him down a ramp in the loading bay when Anita turned around and stopped him.

Anita has tried to find productive avenues for Will's ceaseless energy, such as swimming and gymnastics, but Will has been too disruptive and, while ashamed to admit it, Anita has been very embarrassed by his behaviour. Their home life has become very tense and stressful. Anita is often in tears and the times that John is home, they often argue, usually over the management of Will's behaviour.

Anita has contemplated reducing her hours, or even giving up work altogether, to spend more time with her children, and she wonders where she has gone

➤

case study

wrong in her parenting. However, Anita is very good at her work and her success in part helps to make up for her feelings of inadequacy as a mother; at least she can control her work day.

Last week, Anita met with Will's teacher who said that Will had been disruptive in class, his standard of work had been poor and he didn't seem able to concentrate. Will's teacher suggested that Anita take Will to be assessed by their family doctor because of his behavioural problems. Anita was very confronted by this because she didn't want to admit to people outside their immediate family that there might be something wrong with Will. She felt that she was failing in her job as a mother and she didn't want others to know. At the same time, she was also keen to find out whether there might be something wrong with Will and perhaps it wasn't just her parenting after all. If there was nothing wrong, then the blame for his behaviour would rest with her.

She was in a quandary but eventually decided to take Will to the doctor. After listening to her concerns about Will's behaviour and conducting a physical examination, the doctor concluded that he most likely did have attention deficit hyperactivity disorder (ADHD). He explained that he could prescribe Ritalin, which would alleviate the symptoms of this disorder—hyperactivity, inattention and impulsiveness. Anita was both shocked and relieved: shocked to learn that there really was something medically wrong with Will and relieved to learn that something could be done about it—perhaps it wasn't all her fault after all?

Questions

1   How would biomedical and sociological approaches differ in their explanations for the situation in the case study? What factors would they emphasise?
2   How do the concepts of 'social control', 'medicalisation', 'iatrogenesis' and 'victim blaming' help to understand what is happening in the case study?
3   What are the dominant discourses around families, parenting, education and medicine that are evident in the case study?
4   Who benefits most from the solution that is provided in the case study?
5   How can we determine whether something is 'bad behaviour' or a 'symptom'? What is the difference?

This case study provides an example of medicalisation of the behaviour of children. Hyperkinesis has a long history but the history of attention deficit hyperactivity disorder (ADHD) is much shorter. Originally hyperkinesis did not have any definitive biological causes; however, it manifested in children over the age of five who were overactive, impulsive and easily distracted. It was known that the use of amphetamines had a settling effect but because of the highly addictive nature of these drugs and their side effects, they were not readily prescribed to children; however, this changed when Ritalin became available in the 1960s. In the 1980s, when hyperkinesis became known as attention deficit hyperactivity disorder, this broadened the category of patient from predominantly boys to include girls, all ages and a broader range of 'attention' related symptoms.

Thus, the pressure to prescribe and use Ritalin also came from teachers and parents who not only wanted to improve the child's behaviour but also to shift the blame from their teaching or parenting ability to the child's disease. In this instance, medicalisation has been used as a tool to enhance the success of the child, the mother and the teacher. As Singh (2004: 1204) argues, 'The problem is that a pill promotes medications and an obscuring of the cultural components of both "behavioural disorder" and "good mothering"'.

TO TRUE! over prescribed

CONCLUSION

While it is clear that biomedicine has made significant contributions to our knowledge, understanding and treatment of illness and disease, a sociological approach to understanding biomedicine illustrates how knowledge, power and discourse are intertwined. The aim of this chapter has not been to suggest that we should discard the biomedical model. Clearly, a good dose of sociological theory will not suffice as a treatment for a bleeding wound or coronary artery disease. However, the contribution of sociology to our understanding of health and illness is to critically examine the knowledge claims that may be made about illness, critique the dominance of a single approach and point to alternative ways of understanding health and illness in the population.

REVIEW QUESTIONS

1   What discourses are privileged in debates about asthma, HIV-AIDS and cancer? How does this shape approaches to these illnesses? What other discourses may exist?
2   What is meant by the claim that scientific knowledge is socially constructed? How does this affect our understanding of medical knowledge?
3   Are the benefits that medicine brings to our society outweighed by the 'side effects' of the biomedical approach?
4   Can you think of a time when you were feeling unwell, but the scientific medical tests that were conducted failed to find anything abnormal? What reason was given for your illness in the absence of scientific evidence?

KEY TERMS

Biomedicine/biomedical model
Discourse/dominant discourse
Iatrogenesis/cascade iatrogenesis
Legitimacy
Medicalisation

Paradigm
Randomised control trial
Social control
Truth
Victim blaming

FURTHER READING

Barry, A.M. and Yuill, C. 2002, *Understanding Health: A Sociological Introduction*, London, Sage.

Cheek, J., Shoebridge, J., Willis, E. and Zadoroznyj, M. 1996, *Society and Health, Social Theory for Health Workers*, Melbourne, Longman.

Conrad, P. 1992, 'Medicalization and social control', *Annual Review of Sociology*, 18, pp. 209–32.

Illich, I. 1976, *Limits to Medicine: Medical Nemesis, the Expropriation of Health*, London, Boyars.

Kuhn, T.S. 1962, *The Structure of Scientific Revolutions*, Chicago, University of Chicago Press.

Lupton, D. 2003, *Medicine as Culture*, London, Sage.

Petersen, A.R. 1994, *In a Critical Condition: Health and Power Relations in Australia*, St Leonards, Allen & Unwin.

Chapter 3

Lay, Folk and Consumer Ideas about Health and Illness

Introduction

Julia is starting to recognise that sociological understandings of health and illness involve a process of deconstructing common sense beliefs and thinking about issues from other perspectives. At the beginning of the day's lecture, while Julia was pondering the alternative explanations highlighted over the past week or so, she had a thought. Around her sat different people from a variety of backgrounds—there were women, men, young people and older people; moreover, there were many people from different ethnic backgrounds. Julia assumed that health and illness issues in different countries would be unlike those in Australia. Does this mean that people from different countries have their own knowledge and beliefs about health and illness? By considering the recent point that knowledge is shaped by social, cultural and historical conditions, Julia suddenly became fascinated by how her understanding of health and illness may be different to those held by the people who sat around her in the lecture theatre.

In contemporary Western societies, the field of health is dominated by expert knowledge forms. However, there are other forms of knowledge that exert powerful influences over the experience of health and illness. The power of the biomedical model explored in the previous chapter means that alternative viewpoints are often presented as irrational, thus denying the power of ideas, beliefs and values that are seen as being 'non-orthodox'. Two broad categories can be discerned in studying these approaches to health and illness. First, folk models of health and illness are models of health that are cross-cultural in variation and, in particular, comprise traditional cultural forms of health knowledge. Second, lay health beliefs shape the experience of health within Western cultures. This is sometimes referred to as subcultural research. Most notably, research has examined differences between social classes in health beliefs and, to a lesser extent, gender. More recently, the idea of 'lay epidemiology' has forced a reconsideration about health care ideas and practices, and in particular, about the role of 'lay' consumers in health care.

This chapter aims to extend our understanding of the way in which such ideas inform the health and illness experience. We start by exploring the importance of alternative models of healing, where there is a designated healing modality and, often, designated healers—known in Western cultures as 'folk models' of health and healing. We then explore 'lay' models of health and how lay ideas about health and illness are influential in shaping the illness experience in cultures when biomedicine is the orthodox healing modality. Finally we examine how changing consumer expectations have shaped contemporary health and healing in Western cultures, and how this has shifted the way in which we understand the idea of lay health.

Objectives

After reading this chapter, you should be able to:

■ define and discuss the concepts of lay and folk healing
■ critically evaluate the competing claims to knowledge
■ describe how differing perspectives on health and illness may shape the illness experience
■ explore how ideas about health change over time and within cultures.

Overview of folk and lay approaches

Health is not simply a biological function. It is experienced through our social location and in the ways we live and experience life. Therefore, it stands to reason that there are alternative ways of understanding and responding to illness issues. Kleinman (1988) has argued that in contemporary societies, professional knowledge based on scientific approaches to healing coexists with alternative knowledge forms. Folk models of health draw on cultural knowledges, and their knowledge may be closely linked with 'how to live' within their specific group (i.e. health may be linked with rituals that have a moral or religious value). Popular (or lay) approaches comprise health and illness activities derived from family or community sources. They may draw on both experiential and scientific knowledge when understanding and responding to health and illness issues.

Researchers working in the area of lay and folk ideas about health and illness argue that the language itself contributes to the distancing between the various forms of knowledge where lay and folk models are deemed to be less powerful than professional or orthodox knowledge. Stacey claims that even though the term 'lay' originated in the Greek 'of the people', it tends to be used for those people who do not belong to a specific profession. 'In referring to people who lack particular qualifications … "lay" suggests the absence of something valuable or prestigious, and may imply less competence, or even less moral worth' (Stacey, 1994: 90). Similarly, folk models of healing tend to suggest something that is not scientific, but rather simply a cultural belief and therefore of lesser value. In Western cultures, we tend to view these models from an ethnocentric standpoint— that is, through taking our own position where biomedicine is dominant as the superior way in which we should deal with health and illness problems, and thus judging other models as inferior. However, Pill (1991: 204) argues 'lay [and folk] and professional beliefs are equally products of their own cultures and therefore reflect key preoccupations of the society at that particular time and place'.

The importance of understanding folk and lay knowledges is a recurrent theme through the literature, which is written largely by Western anthropologists, sociologists and health practitioners. This is because it is argued that understanding people's lay or folk perspectives may better inform Western health care and

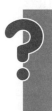

Question for reflection

Migraine is a common health complaint. What are the differing types of knowledge that we may draw on to help understand the causes and treatments for migraine?

health promotion practices. However, it is also argued that we need to look more widely at the differing knowledge forms and see each of them as informing health knowledge and action in an increasingly complex society, in a way that may, or may not, coexist with the ideas within biomedicine and health promotion.

Folk models

Folk healing may be defined as a set of health beliefs and practices derived from ethnic and historical traditions that have the amelioration or cure of psychological, spiritual and physical problems as their goal. These health beliefs are based on the notion that healing is an art that includes culturally appropriate methods of treatment delivered by recognised healers in the community who capitalise on a patient's faith and belief systems in the treatment process (Lozano Applewhite, 1995). One characteristic of folk-healing models is that healing wisdom is often passed through an apprenticeship model of training—whether this be by virtue of birth (where healing is passed through generations) or by some other selection process.

Given the cultural diversity of most Western societies (including Australia), it is important to recognise the significance of folk models of healing for people in our own society. Some folk beliefs may be viewed as therapeutic, harmless and, in some cases, dangerous, as people negotiate their way through a traditional knowledge system in conjunction with Western medical knowledge. There may be high variation in the explanations that are provided for health and illness, whether these are related to superstition or magic, social and cultural practices, or systematic bodies of healing knowledge.

The following section provides some examples of folk models of healing. While there is an extreme diversity of folk healing (any Internet search will provide you with a seemingly limitless catalogue), these examples highlight key issues of interest in understanding the influence of these models. First, these systems have a healer who has a distinctive role to play in the healing process; second, we need to be mindful that models of healing are not static and indeed the same underlying model may have geographic or cultural variation; and third, like culture, models of healing may adapt and change, and may coexist alongside other forms of healing, such as biomedicine. For example, Lopez (2005) describes contemporary Mexican folk medicine as a blending of native American Indian religions and Roman Catholic ideas about healing and illness as being 'God's will', showing that explanatory frameworks change according to the influence of new ideas that take on significance within the wider cultural setting. From a sociological perspective, we are interested in these models as an authoritative knowledge form—authority may be vested in the role of the healer, a wider view of the world (i.e. in gods and moral values), and the routine practices that make up the components of the folk model.

Example one: traditional Chinese medicine

An analysis of traditional Chinese medicine illustrates that folk models can be complex knowledge forms. Healing according to this model occurs in a context emphasising the significance of the social being, ethical relationships and interdependence (Kao et al., 2006). In such a system, concepts such as blood building are critical to understanding health measures within Chinese culture. Three concepts that dominated ancient Chinese philosophy and medicine— the Tao, the yin and yang, and the five elements (wood, fire, earth, metal and water)—are interwoven into beliefs about blood-building foods. The Tao is the abstract motivator and moral guide that brought order out of chaos when the world was created. This was done by dividing the two opposing forces, yin (female, negative, dark and cold) and yang (male, positive, light and warm). A balance between yin and yang is necessary for healthy blood circulation as well as for adequate vital energy. This is often seen as a balance between hot and cold. Menstruation, parturition and the post-partum period are yin conditions during which a woman has 'too much coldness' and her blood is believed to be thickened. Protein-rich soups containing such ingredients as chicken, pork liver, eggs, pig's feet or oxtail are particularly important 'hot tonics' that are often prescribed. Some specific food combinations are also believed to help flush out dirty blood during the post-partum period. There are also combinations of foods for body building. The selection and frequency of consumption of tonic soups and herbal teas vary with geographic availability of ingredients, regional and family custom, economic ability, degree of adherence to cultural practices and traditional beliefs, and amount deemed necessary to restore balance (Ludman et al., 1989). This then is a very complex folk medicine system.

Example two: interactions between Western and folk models of healing

Folk health beliefs may interact with Western medicine, with consumers using both methods, as they deem appropriate. Using the example of Mexican Americans, Lopez (2005) points to three coexisting explanations for this. The first (in response to the introduction of Spanish ideas) represents 'Western' ideas about illness at an historical time when Hippocratic theories focused on attaining a proper balance of the body's four humours—hot fluids of blood and yellow bile, and cold fluids of phlegm and black bile. Second, and also an explanation that focuses on imbalance, are the ideas of 'bad airs'—with the focus on certain conditions being defined by exposure to hot or cold conditions. Third, is the impact of spiritual and socio-personal imbalances. These are the most feared and many relate to what Western medicine would term potential mental illness. Transmitted as a result of personal transgression or by 'supernatural hex', these can include 'headaches, fever, or even death' (Lopez, 2005: 25). Other interpersonal illnesses such as 'susto' and 'espanto' relate to 'soul loss' or 'loss of spirit', which cause depression, physical weakness and apathy, the cause often being related to extreme fright or trauma, with death being an outcome if it is left untreated.

A study of elderly Mexican Americans found that while many had been exposed to the expertise of various folk healers during childhood, and had used them for childhood illnesses, they tended to use both Western and folk practitioners, drawing on medicine, traditional healing and religion in their explanations for illness and treatment choices. For mild illnesses, they tended to believe that herbal remedies were appropriate, either by self-medicating or seeking a folk healer. The power of God and the faith in God's will was a powerful way in which they expressed dissatisfaction with both Western and folk medicine. Recognising that traditional healers (*curanderos*) may have the gift of healing, and that medical doctors may have education, they argued that ultimately it was the divine will of God that enabled a cure to be effected (Lozano Applewhite, 1995).

Further integration of Western medicine and folk healing occurs in complex ways. Craig's (2000: 710) case study of Vietnamese ideas about health and healing show that while the idea of the 'germ theory' has been recognised among Vietnamese communities, germs are 'widely understood as only being able to penetrate into the boundaries of the body if the body is weak first'. He discusses the ways that folk models of health represent embodied forms of knowledge that are integral to the way in which life is carried out—Western medicine is seen as representing a disembodied form of knowledge. Craig discusses the way in which the rhythms of everyday life are combined with the rhythms of health and healing practices. Again, the significance of hot and cold, environmental factors, and boundaries between inside the body and outside the body become important in understanding illness. Craig also argues that there is a 'practical logic' to the knowledge and practice that sees the act of healing and the emotional and nurturing response as equally important in healing practices. Consider the example he gives:

> Remedies like rubbing Vicks cut with coconut oil onto the back of a child who is having difficulty breathing, or the similar Vietnamese remedy of 'beating the wind' (*danh gio*, a massage with mentholated oil and perhaps a coin), are a regular part of daily care … Having such a massage performed is more than just a medical treatment: it is a warm and deeply memorable part of family and friend's nurture. (Craig, 2000: 708)

Example three: health in Australian Indigenous cultures

In Australian society, Indigenous traditions have their own models of health and healing that can powerfully shape the illness experience. Belief systems that attribute a powerful role to supernatural interventions help to explain the distribution of illness and death, as well as having important social control functions within Aboriginal societies. Thus, belief systems about health are intricately connected with other aspects of life such as the land, kinship obligations and religion, with an emphasis on the importance of harmony in all of these in order to maintain health within the individual (Maher, 1999: 230). The focus on the supernatural and the role of sorcery is one reason that Gray argues that the healing system of the Yolngu people in north-east Arnhem Land is a 'personalistic' one—so named because 'of the belief that all illnesses are caused by the purposeful intervention of an active agent' (Gray, 2006: 238). However, many mild illnesses are not given this explanation; instead a naturalistic explanation locates illness as a disruption to bodily equilibrium or balance (Gray, 2006: 238). In these cases remedies are found in traditional bush medicine, rather than through the intervention of a healer with magical or supernatural powers.

Although healing specialists exist in Indigenous cultures, knowledge of healing is more diffuse than we experience in Western society—where power is vested in a medical practitioner—particularly where there is a combination of personalistic and naturalistic explanations for illness. Among the Yolngu people, the specialist healer receives their healing capacity through a spiritual experience, the evidence for which must then be demonstrated to other tribe members (Gray, 2006: 241). More broadly, knowledge is better encapsulated as 'family' or 'community' knowledge that is passed through ritual; 'yarning', a key component of which is respect; and an illustrative tradition of relating knowledge to the local environment and to spiritual beliefs (Craig, 2000). This is in clear contrast to the reductionism of biomedicine. The holism of Indigenous health beliefs emphasises connection to the land, cultural rituals and each other are essential for healing. One notable factor (found in other folk models and cultures as well) is the clear-cut boundary between women's and men's business in healing. These boundaries prescribe certain roles and responsibilities in the wider community, as well as in matters of healing (Maher, 1999: 232). The importance of such boundary maintenance can be seen in the rituals around reproductive matters, which bring together both health and cultural knowledge.

All these examples highlight the ways culture and healing are intermixed—emphasising that health practices are inextricably linked to the social and cultural relations within differing cultural groups. Thus, the definition of disease found in societies that emphasise biomedical healing model is at odds with the cultural understanding of disease found in many non-Western societal groups. What must also be noted in contemporary society is that ideas of folk healing are not static, but change when interacting with other models of healing or social influences.

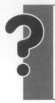

Question for reflection

Drawing on the examples above, what do you see as the defining characteristics of folk models of healing?

Lay models of health and disease

Lay models are models of health and illness that clearly coexist with the dominant orthodox approach. When referring to lay models, we are generally referring to those beliefs about health that are not reliant upon an alternative healing system, as is the case with most folk models. Lay models represent 'people wisdom' about health and illness, rather than an organised way of dealing with the illness experience that is found in folk models. The distinction is, of course, blurred. What characterises lay models of health is that they are informal, experiential and mostly unwritten (Stacey, 1994), compared to the systematic scientific approach of professional knowledge. However, there is often an integration of experiential and scientific knowledge in lay accounts of health and illness. And, as Furnham (1994: 716) notes, 'these beliefs form a "system" in the sense that they are interconnected to other non-illness related beliefs, but also because they are connected to the beliefs of other people in the community'.

There is some debate about whether people can be 'lay experts' (Prior, 2003), and whether discussion of lay perspectives should focus on 'lay accounts' rather than giving them the title of 'beliefs'. For example, Shaw (2002) argues that because many common sense understandings are based on the dominant expert paradigm of thinking, they are thus accounts of illness rather than distinct belief systems. MacDougall (2003) uses the term 'ordinary theories' to denote ideas that differ from, complement or challenge expert theories. He argues that both experts and 'ordinary people' engage in thinking about, constructing and testing ideas about illness, explanations and solutions. His study examined ideas about fitness and found that while people incorporated 'expert' opinion into their ideas about the importance of fitness, they also drew on other sources of knowledge. For example, he identified a 'reservoir theory'—the idea that the body has a finite capacity for exercise, and therefore one must be careful about not overusing it. Thus 'people listen to their body, make trade-offs and decide how much of the reservoir to use at a particular time' (MacDougall, 2003: 390). This contrasts with the 'more is better' idea that underpins much contemporary professional advice about exercise.

In a classic study of the ideas about colds and flu among patients of a north London general practice, Helman (1978) argued that lay explanations could be identified. Chills and colds related to individual interaction with the natural environment. In this view, damp or rain (cold/wet conditions) or cold winds or draughts (cold/dry) can penetrate the boundary of the skin and cause similar conditions within the body. By contrast, fevers and flu originate in other people and are caused by germs that travel through the air. Patients also classified their illness according to whether they felt hot or cold rather than by any medical definition of colds and fevers.

As with folk systems of healing, there is wide variation in lay beliefs about health, illness and healing. In reviewing research in this area, Hughner and Kleine (2004) identified key ways in which lay health beliefs can be categorised:

1   Definitions of health: while some studies have shown that health is defined as 'absence of disease', others have demonstrated people's emphasis on functionality (a person is healthy if they are able to perform their daily duties), equilibrium and freedom. Thus, whether health is seen as a positive value for living a full and happy life, or a prerequisite for functional survival, varies according to circumstance. Calnan's work on conceptions of health among working-class and middle-class women pointed to different language used by different groups. Whereas middle-class women described health as 'being fit', 'strong' and 'active', working-class women focused more on functional requirements. They emphasised the importance of 'getting through the day' as representing health, along with the concept of 'never being ill' (Calnan, 1987:33).

2   Explaining health/illness and how to maintain good health: an exploration of the literature reveals that people's beliefs often draw on individual explanations in their ideas about why people get sick or how to maintain good health. Such explanations include: the importance of meditation and prayer; having a good mental attitude; that work is a valuable way of staying healthy; belief in religious or supernatural forces; that one has a moral responsibility to take good care of oneself; and the importance of self-monitoring—either hygiene or cleanliness, or regular medical check-ups.

3   Identification of factors that affect health: in contrast to the above category, there is also a range of beliefs about the factors that affect health that are largely outside the control of the individual. Examples include the effect on health by policies and institutions, the environment, and genetics.

Lay models of health are important because they influence health action and illness-seeking behaviour. As well as informing what action will be taken (this can range from folk cures, other forms of self-medication and specific actions ranging from bed rest to brisk exercise), lay beliefs also dictate who people turn to for advice when they become ill. Furnham (1994) cites research indicating that people seek information from a range of people (family, other people with similar illness experience, paramedics or other service providers who deal with the public, self-help and religious sources) with advisors' credentials based more on experience than on formal medical status or specific medical expertise.

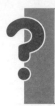

Questions for reflection

Which lay health practices do you participate in? Which lay beliefs or practices do you think are completely illogical? Why?

Knowing about health patterns: scientific, social and lay epidemiology

While lay beliefs are important in understanding health knowledge, the scientific approach to studying the incidence and prevalence of disease is epidemiology. Last (1995: 55) defines epidemiology as 'the study of the distribution and determinants of health-related states or events in specified populations, and the application of this study to the control of health problems'. Epidemiology provides information about causal links such as smoking and lung disease, obesity and diabetes, or alcohol consumption and hypertension. These causal links are often the basis for health promotion messages that encourage individuals to make healthy lifestyle choices. A criticism of epidemiological approaches has been the fact that they are more likely to focus on the disease, reflecting their origins as a medical specialty primarily concerned with cure rather than prevention and thus firmly embedded in the biomedical model.

See Chapter 5

Epidemiology relies heavily on demographic data that describe the compositions of populations, such as overall size of populations and variables such as age, sex, housing, tenure, employment status, areas of residence, household and family size, and female fertility patterns. Baum (2002) argues that epidemiological studies can provide the links between various risk factors, but are unlikely to provide convincing evidence on their own. A number of studies are needed to document causality. For example, the link between tobacco smoking and lung cancer only gained credibility as more and more studies provided proof of the relationship.

Taking a sociological view of health is consistent with a form of epidemiology known as social epidemiology, which focuses on studies describing and explaining diseases in *whole* populations. Social epidemiology differs from mainstream epidemiology because it seeks to understand why social groups are more or less healthy, rather than focusing on individuals (Kawachi, 2002). In this way, social epidemiology tries to uncover why some societies have higher rates of diabetes, obesity or hypertension by examining the social determinants of health. Like traditional forms of epidemiology, social epidemiology is concerned with establishing causal links; however, the associations are between social factors and population health (Kawachi, 2002).

In contrast, the concept of 'lay epidemiology' explains the distribution of health and illness, *as experienced or perceived by those people who are affected*. Lay epidemiology is defined as 'a scheme in which individuals interpret health risks through the routine observation and discussion of cases of illness and death in personal networks and in the public arena as well as from formal and informal evidence arising from other sources, such as television and magazines' (Frankel et al., 1991: 428). Lay epidemiology, then, draws on the knowledge that may be shared across generations and situated within communities. People seek to explain occurrences of illness through their own experiences and the 'lore' they share with others. The terminology has shifted from lay health beliefs (the concept of beliefs suggests that they can be modified or changed) to lay epidemiology (suggesting that lay health ideas, beliefs and values actually constitute 'knowledge'). The term 'lay epidemiology' thus provides a more legitimate and authoritative term for those knowledge forms that sit outside formal, 'scientific' knowledge. The experiential knowledge of lay epidemiology has been used when people have identified 'unproven' causes of ill health—either through exposure to toxic environments, unsafe workplace environments, or the side effects of drug treatments (Popay & Williams, 1996). In cases such as these, scientific evidence may be unable, or slow, to 'prove causality', yet the experiential knowledge that is accumulated may demonstrate clearly adverse impacts on health. It is therefore important to understand a person's world view, rather than just objective health information.

Issues around lifestyle have emerged as important areas of contestation between professional and lay knowledges. With information derived from scientific epidemiological studies, lifestyle is 'a concept which has come to refer to people's styles of living which, in turn, are shaped by their patterns of consumption' (Nettleton, 1995: 37). The dominant approach to the increasing number of people with risk factors for lifestyle diseases is to require compliance with medical advice. Such advice may include drug therapy, exercise regimes and dietary changes. However, while medical advice on the avoidance of the risks to health posed by an unhealthy lifestyle is seemingly straightforward, the integration of this advice into people's lives when they draw on differing frameworks of understanding complicates the extent to which 'lifestyle advice' provides a meaningful set of actions.

Further, experiential knowledge confounds medical knowledge based on epidemiology. In many cases, disease is seen as random, which runs counter to epidemiological evidence or even to much social scientific evidence. In particular, people may draw on fatalistic explanations in their understanding of health and illness, contradicting official accounts that focus on lifestyle modification and risk factors. While medical advice may be seemingly straightforward, it is possible to cite cases where people 'who had very "good" lifestyles had fatal heart attacks at an early age while others who had very "bad" lifestyles lived to a ripe old age' (Wiles, 1998: 1482). This leads to the conclusion that heart attacks are the result of fate and forces outside the control of individuals, rather than amenable to their own control through lifestyle. The way that health experts place lifestyle at the centre of their theory of disease causation, and thereby de-emphasise other aspects that contribute to health and illness, is also critiqued by lay epidemiologists. As Davison et al. (1992: 683) say, 'Falling back on the albeit honest defence that lifestyle advice is based on probability rather than certainty is plainly an inadequate response when the complexities of popular culture are properly taken into consideration'. They point to a range of other factors that may be important: personal attributes (heredity, upbringing and personal traits); social environment (wealth, resources, risks associated with occupation, etc.); the physical environment (climate, natural dangers, environmental contamination); and ideas around luck, chance and the random nature of illness (Davison et al., 1992: 679).

Research focusing on ideas of control in a lower socio-economic group by Bolam et al. (2003) found that people emphasised both fatalistic beliefs and the need to think (and act) positively in their approaches to health. It is argued that such seemingly contradictory views on health are also reflective of broader debates about structure and agency. The interweaving of beliefs in both fate and positive thinking is, according to Bolam et al. (2003: 26), an attempt to 'try and resolve the tension between them, demonstrating a motivation to remain positive whilst acknowledging material and other restraints on one's ability to take control'. Confronted with the experiential evidence, based on personal experience, lifestyle change may not be viewed as a rational action.

As can be seen, the issue of non-compliance with medical advice is contentious. Medical compliance has been defined as 'the extent to which the patient's behavior (in terms of taking medications, following diets, or executing other lifestyle changes) coincides with medical or health advice' (Trostle, 1988: 1299). However, as studies of people with heart disease (Wiles, 1998) and diabetes (Schoenberg et al., 1998) demonstrate, there is not a straightforward translation of scientific health advice into individual health action. As Trostle claims, non-compliance is an unavoidable by-product of collisions between the clinical world and other competing worlds of work, play, friendship and family life. The beliefs that people bring to their situation may result in a range of actions, from compliance with medical advice, through to total non-compliance. Many people partially comply with health advice, suggesting that there is a complex interplay between one's social situation, health beliefs and adoption of medical knowledge.

Question for reflection

Is there any common ground between scientific epidemiology and lay epidemiology? Give reasons for your answer.

Consumers and the challenge to expertise

Further, even if no dissent or contestation is evident, it is argued by sociologists of science such as Wynne (1996: 50) that people 'informally but incessantly problematise their own relationships with expertise of all kinds'. This has been seen in health care with the rise of a 'consumer movement' that has focused attention on the need for consumers to have greater information, rights to appropriate services and protection from high costs of care. A key component of the consumer movement is the sharing of knowledge and information. This shifts the experience of health care from an individualised encounter to one that identifies discrepancies in practice and information provision. It locates consumers as people who are affected by their position in society, experiences of illness and medical care. Lay health consumers are active and critical, have a complex belief system about health and health care, knowledge of one's health requirements, and are discerning in the use of professional medical expertise (Calnan, 1987). Lay models of health are therefore a challenge to the idea of the patient who is represented as passive and subservient in the health care encounter. The health consumer exercises rights and choice. It has been suggested that such a shift in capacity to exercise power has resulted in the 'deprofessionalisation' of health (Irvine, 1999: 182) due to greater access to education and information, and the capacity to make choices about the type of health care provider. Where once the doctor may have been the sole source of information, contemporary health consumers are encouraged to access further information about other available services, side effects of medication and other health-promoting behaviours (Irvine, 2002: 35).

Undeniably, the rise of the 'information society' has been an integral tool for greater consumer participation in health care decision making and access to alternative health beliefs and models. That such information exists on a massive scale, and may be competing and/or contradictory, is the consequence of living in an 'information-rich society'. Such information requires considerable skills in accessing and negotiating (Hardey, 1999: 821)—a far cry from reliance on a system that privileges a single, expert voice. Indeed, it is argued that medical autonomy and its claims as the sole source of expert knowledge is likely to be undermined by the use of information through sources such as the Internet. Hardey (1999: 828) claims that this is not dissimilar to the diversity of voices that existed in the health market prior to the ascendency of the medical profession. And while it is conceded that the dominant form of health knowledge in Western societies is biomedical knowledge, it must be acknowledged that the diversity of information available enables the blurring of the orthodox and non-orthodox in a way that 'encourages a definition of health that embraces spiritual and emotional dimensions often marginal in conventional medicine' (Hardey, 1999: 832). The Internet is discussed further in the next chapter.

case study

One of Julia's class mates, Andy, is a 22-year-old male who grew up in a quiet rural area on the outskirts of Hobart, Tasmania. His parents operate an organic apple orchard and both of his sisters have started an organic herb market garden on the same property. Andy's dad went to university to study agricultural science and now Andy has enrolled as a nursing student. His mother studied to be a librarian a long time ago, but the organics market has increased in demand so she now co-manages the orchard with Andy's dad. Andy's family are very health conscious people who exercise regularly.

Andy, in particular, loves to run. He participates in marathons and fun runs, and trains every day just to keep fit. Recently Andy has noticed that a vein in the back of his leg has started to protrude and changed colour to a darkish blue. He has felt some unusual aching in this area when sitting for long periods of time in class and it hasn't been improved by his daily training regimen. His mum thinks it's a healthy sign that lots of blood is pumping through his veins as a result of his active lifestyle and exercising; 'We eat such healthy food and maintain an active pace', said his mum, 'You can't possibly have anything wrong with you'. But the aching hasn't stopped, so Andy visited his general practitioner (GP).

Andy's GP diagnosed Andy with a varicose vein on the back of his leg—probably from the strain of running in combination with sitting for long periods of time in the classroom. She refers him to a phlebologist (a vein specialist) and also asks to book him in for an ultrasound just in case there is a blood clot. But Andy doesn't understand why he has to pay so much money for treatment when really he is an active person who always maintains his health. At university the next day, Andy searches the Internet for some more information about vein health with the aim of finding some alternative treatment options to those offered by his GP. There is a great deal of information available on many websites, which he finds really useful. Finally, Andy decides to give running a miss for a week or so until the pain stops, and he visits his local health food shop for some horse chestnut seed extract, which his mum said will reduce the swelling if he does have a varicose vein.

Questions

1   What knowledge influenced the health action taken by Andy and his mum? Do you think he made the right choice?
2   Which model of health and illness informed the treatment recommended by Andy's GP?
3   What was it about Andy's decisions after his GP's diagnosis that locates him as a 'lay health consumer'?
4   Can you think of a time when you may have acted in a similar way to Andy? Recall why you made these choices and how you went about getting alternative advice. Did you use the Internet? What other sources of information did you seek out? Do you think other people would necessarily follow the same action? Why or why not?

case study

CONCLUSION

Folk and lay approaches to health and illness present different knowledge forms to those of biomedicine. While folk health models draw on magic and supernatural forces, they also coexist with expert knowledges. Lay health beliefs are an important way in which we can understand 'why people do what they do', even though their actions may seem to be contradictory to expert knowledge. As health professionals, it is important to be aware of these differing approaches to health and illness, as they shape health practices and actions, and may powerfully influence the illness experience. These ideas are not static, they change as social conditions change. They may coexist with, or contradict, scientific epidemiological information. The rise of the health care consumer also focuses attention on the ways in which the provision of health care must adapt to changing circumstances.

REVIEW QUESTIONS

1   Do a Google search of folk models of healing. What are the characteristics of the models you find? Do they have a designated healer? Who is the healer and where does their authority to heal come from?

2   Consider the lay ideas you grew up with—sometimes known as 'old wives tales'. You may have had particular ideas about health and illness, and particular remedies for health complaints. Compare your 'experiential wisdom' with other students. How can you assess which is the most valid?

3   Why don't people always follow health advice?

4   What is the role of the 'lay' consumer in health care systems dominated by a biomedical approach? How might lay ideas about health constrain or enable medical authority?

KEY TERMS

Consumer/consumer movement

Culture

Deprofessionalisation

Epidemiology, lay epidemiology,
    social epidemiology

Ethnocentric

Folk models

Information society

Lay health beliefs

Lifestyle

Medical autonomy

Non-compliance

Personalistic/naturalistic

Structure/agency

FURTHER READING

Calnan, M. 1987, *Health and Illness: A Lay Perspective*, London, Tavistock.

Davison, C., Frankel, S. and Davey Smith, G. 1992, 'The limits of lifestyle: re-assessing "fatalism" in the popular culture of illness prevention', *Social Science & Medicine*, 34, pp. 675–85.

Gray, D.E. 2006, *Health Sociology: An Australian Perspective*, Frenchs Forest, Pearson Education.

Helman, C. 1978, '"Feed a cold, starve a fever": folk models of infection in an English suburban community, and their relation to medical treatment', *Culture, Medicine and Psychiatry*, 2, pp. 107–37.

Hughner, R.S. and Kleine, S.S. 2004, 'Views of health in the lay sector: a compilation and review of how individuals think about health', *Health: An Interdisciplinary Journal for the Social Study of Health, Illness and Medicine*, 8, pp. 395–422.

Kleinman, A. 1988, *The Illness Narratives: Suffering, Healing and the Human Condition*, New York, Basic Books.

Maher, P. 1999, 'A review of "traditional" Aboriginal health beliefs', *Australian Journal of Rural Health*, 7, pp. 229–36.

Nettleton, S. 1995, *The Sociology of Health and Illness*, Cambridge, Polity Press.

Popay, J. and Williams, G. (eds) 1994, *Researching the People's Health*, London, Routledge.

Chapter 4

The Media and Health

Introduction

What do we mean by the media? Media is a shortened version of the term media communication, which refers to organised ways of disseminating information, opinions and entertainment. O'Shaughnessy and Stadler (2005: 3) define the media as 'the media industry and the communication technologies involved in transmitting information and entertainment between senders and receivers across space and time'. The term mass media refers to the section of the media designed to reach large audiences. The primary media for mass communication are publishing (newspapers, magazines and books), broadcasting (radio and television) and film (cinema, DVD and video). Mass communication is traditionally a one-way process with relatively few senders of messages and a great many receivers of messages. This is changing with the introduction of new 'interactive' media, such as the Internet and the World Wide Web.

This chapter explores the different forms of media and the issue of media ownership. This discussion draws our attention to the ability of the mass media to pervasively and powerfully shape our understanding of the social world. We then turn our focus to the ways in which the media construct ideas and meanings about health and illness. We argue that it is important for health professionals in contemporary society to understand the role of the media for two reasons: first, to be able to critically explore the influence of the media on our own understanding of health and illness; and second, to understand how the health and illness experiences of others are shaped by the media.

Objectives

After reading this chapter, you should be able to:

- describe the way that mass media contributes to our understanding of the social world
- understand the differing ways that health information is both portrayed in and retrieved from the media
- critically analyse the construction of meaning in media text.

The media

Mass media include print media (newspapers, magazines and journals, books, advertising) and electronic media (television, radio, film–video and cinema). Increasingly, we are seeing the influence of new information technologies (the Internet). Australia is one of the biggest consumers of communication and information technology in the world. In 2000, 99 per cent of Australian households had a TV; 78 per cent had a VCR; 30 per cent had a mobile phone (the second-highest per capita rate of ownership in the world); 53 per cent had a computer; and 33 per cent (or 1.9 million households) had access to the Internet (Holmes, Hughes & Julian, 2003: 439). This is the fifth-highest density in the world.

Statistics reveal the pervasive influence of mass media over our leisure time. The average Australian watches three hours and 13 minutes of television each day. The over-55 age group watches more—on average four hours and 24 minutes a day. As a result, the average Australian will spend nine years of their life watching television, of which two years and three months are advertisements (Holmes, Hughes & Julian, 2003: 440). Van Krieken et al. (2000: 551) observe: 'When we take into account the shortening working life, these figures mean that over the life course from childhood to old age, Australians spend more time watching television than in paid employment'.

Increasingly, media are becoming interactive. Rather than being passive recipients viewing, reading and listening to media, audience participation is becoming embedded into programming (for example, voting on and off as in *Big Brother*, or *Australian Idol*). An emerging and important form of media is the Internet—a media form where information is 'mass' in that it is open to a global audience, but individuated because there is a requirement to choose from limitless options. Internet forums, blogs and MSN also have significantly changed how individuals communicate using these media technologies.

The Internet is one of the fastest-growing technologies in history. In just a few brief years, the Internet has moved from being a medium for a small elite group of researchers, 'techies' and 'geeks', and countercultural communities to a medium commonly used by ordinary people. The Internet has become a part of everyday life and transformed the way we conduct business, politics and governance. It has profoundly reshaped our culture. At the end of 2001, it was estimated that there were over 500 million Internet users worldwide, up from 16 million in 1996 (Castells, 2002). In 1995, five years after it first became widely available in Australia, only 5 per cent of Australian homes were connected to the Internet. Over the next five years this figure increased more than ten-fold so that by 2001, 53% of households were connected (Holmes, Hughes & Julian, 2003: 455). The growth in Internet usage in Australia increased by 115 per cent from 2000 to 2005 (Internet World, 2006).

Barr (2000: 118) identifies the following types of interactions possible on the Internet:

- one-to-one messaging (e.g. email)
- one-to-many messaging (e.g. listserv)
- distributed message databases (e.g. USENET news group)
- real-time communication (e.g. Internet relay chat (IRC))
- real-time remote computer utilisation (e.g. 'telnet')
- remote information retrieval (e.g. the World Wide Web).

Unlike print and broadcast media, the Internet is a point-to-point communication network, which means that it is capable of connecting people in a two-way dialogue or what Castells (2002: xxxi) describes as 'self-directed, horizontal communication'. The Internet can be described as an anarchic, decentred system because no one individual or group is able to dominate it. Therefore, it is difficult to control and censor the flow of information. As a result, the Internet is 'hailed as a technology that can deliver the "global village", the Internet is trumpeted as a medium that allows for democratised processes not previously possible in the era of broadcast' (Holmes, Hughes & Julian, 2003: 455). Castells (2002) uses the term 'network society' to characterise contemporary social organisation based on these anarchic information networks powered by microelectronic-based information technology.

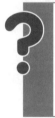

Questions for reflection

What are the advantages and disadvantages of contemporary media? To what extent do contemporary media feature as a characteristic of your everyday life, particularly your interactions with others?

The media and media ownership

From the previous discussion, the pervasive nature of the mass media in our everyday lives is clearly evident and provides us with almost unlimited access to information on an apparently limitless array of topics. This raises questions about who makes this information available and why. It would be reasonable to assume that with access to such a broad range of media in Australia there would be an equally diverse range of opinions. Certainly the Australian Government's Australian Communication and Media Authority objectives, as detailed in the *Broadcasting Services Act 1992*, include the desirability of program diversity, limits on concentration of ownership and foreign control of the mass media, and the need for media to help foster an Australian cultural identity, report news fairly and respect community standards (Australian Communications and Media Authority, 2006). This section draws our attention to the hotly contested issue of media ownership in Australia and the impact this has on the fair and equitable dissemination of information.

The mass media are big business and a normal feature of a capitalist market. It is important to remember that the media are operated as profit-driven businesses. We are familiar with paying to go to the cinema, buying a new CD, the newspaper or our favourite magazine, and renting a DVD, but free-to air television and radio are beamed into our homes at no cost. Who pays? Essentially radio and television use their programs (the 'bait' if you like) to attract audiences who are then sold to advertisers. There are ratings and circulation 'wars' between major competitors to attract the largest audience share, especially during peak viewing times of 6.00 pm to 9.30 pm, so that the station can sell its advertising at a higher fee. The cover price of the newspapers or magazines you buy is also heavily subsidised by advertising.

Australia has one of the highest concentrations of media ownership in the world. Newspaper ownership in Australia's capital cities is dominated by just two corporations, News Limited and John Fairfax Holdings. The largest media owner in Australia is Publishing and Broadcasting Limited (PBL). There is a complex web of relationships between the various media companies. There are close affiliations between particular newspapers, TV stations and radio services. In a democracy, it is argued that citizens need access to accurate information and a forum for debate to raise awareness about important issues, to consider options and eventually to build consensus about appropriate actions. It is in the democratic interests of informed citizens to be able to participate effectively in public debates on issues of importance to them. In theory, the media should provide this role. However, to fulfil this role the media must maintain their independence from the state and all other powerful vested interests. Arguably, this is difficult to achieve in an environment where media ownership is dominated by so few.

The concentration of media ownership is problematic in three main areas. First, for the general public, it means there are less diverse opinions and voices available. Second, this concern is amplified for people in minority or marginalised groups, as they have far fewer opportunities to find a voice and ensure their views reach the public. The third area is related to the absence of healthy market-based competition, which has the potential to decrease the amount of innovation and increase prices.

Prior to 2006, there were strict cross-media ownership laws to prevent one owner from having a monopoly over more than one type of media, and limits to foreign ownership of media outlets. These rules prevented individuals from having a controlling interest in a major daily newspaper *and* a television or radio station serving the same market; however, changes to the legislation in 2006 have relaxed these restrictions. The concentration of media ownership in Australia has not gone unnoticed. Reporters Without Borders compiles an annual Worldwide Press Freedom Index based on press freedom violations such as censorship, regulation of media, arrests of journalists and punishment of press law offences. When the Index was first compiled in 2002, Australia was ranked in twelfth position but had slipped to thirty-fifth place in the 2006 Index after being ranked thirty-first in 2005. Issues identified by Reporters Without Borders as affecting Australia's position on the Index relate to the concentration of media ownership, policies

TABLE 4.1   Worldwide Press Freedom Index 2006

Ranking	Country	Score
1	Finland	0.50
2	Iceland	0.50
3	Ireland	0.50
4	Netherlands	0.50
5	Czech Republic	0.75
6	Estonia	2.00
7	Norway	2.00
8	Slovakia	2.50
9	Switzerland	2.50
10	Hungary	3.00
15	Sweden	4.00
18	Canada	4.50
20	Denmark	5.00
21	New Zealand	5.00
28	United Kingdom	6.50
30	Cyprus	7.50
35	Australia	9.00
44	South Africa	11.25
50	Israel	12.00
56	United States of America	13.00

Excerpt from Worldwide Press Freedom Index 2006, Reporters Without Borders, www.rsf.org

restricting press access to refugees and new anti-terrorist laws, which are viewed as potentially dangerous for journalists (Reporters Without Borders, 2006).

Media ownership may also be important in determining what is reported, the extent of reporting and how long a story remains on the front pages of newspapers and magazines. One of the ways in which the media can influence our understanding of social events is through agenda setting. Lupton (1993: 142) describes the agenda-setting process as 'a social phenomenon by which an issue begins to receive sharply increased media coverage, which in turn provokes widespread public opinion about the issue and eventually leads to responses by policy-makers'. Press coverage can 'set the stage' for determining whether or not an issue emerges as a social problem, and then serves to shape the definition of the problem in the public debate. This may occur through the provision of extensive coverage or by sensationalising particular aspects of the issue (O'Shaughnessy & Stadler, 2005: 25). Consider how issues such as drug use, crime, youth unemployment, Indigenous issues or refugees in Australia are periodically presented as 'crises' in the media, then possibly debated and discussed for a brief period, and then lapse as attention moves to another issue.

Question for reflection

Think of a recent health issue in the media. How do you think this issue was brought to media attention?

The authority of news media

A further reason for exploring the exertion of power in news and entertainment media is the authoritative way in which media are regarded. In the selection of what is deemed 'newsworthy' at any one time, media processes that exclude certain issues or ideas from the public discourse are pivotal, but often not explicitly acknowledged. When an event is labelled as 'news', it carries with it some legitimacy that it is 'reality'. The news media have the weight of 'expert' opinion, and 'fact'. The coverage is often supported with photographs or footage, which reinforce the factual, incontrovertible truth of the story. The notion that the journalists will always portray an unbiased and balanced account of any issue makes it less likely that people will question the representation of issues in the news. In these ways, the news media amass truth value, which tends to render people susceptible to uncritically accepting whatever is presented in the news (unless, of course, they have a vested interest themselves and feel that the interests of their particular group are poorly, inaccurately or unfairly represented).

The line between news that is in the *public interest* and news that has *vested interests* is blurry. Newscasters have immense pressures to produce large volumes of news within space and time constraints. Increasingly they are coming to rely upon outside sources for information that is repackaged and constructed as news, substantially changing the role of the journalist. While the use of news syndicates (e.g. AAP, Reuters) is widely accepted, some would argue this practice eliminates journalists from journalism. More recently, the growth of marketing and public relations has led to an increase in the way that product promotions are repackaged as 'news'. Sometimes these are disclosed as 'infomercials' or 'advertorials', but in other cases there is no declaration of vested interests. The importance of product and consumption is particularly significant in the health market where new ideas and innovations are at a premium for news coverage.

In coverage of issues, the media play an important role in determining who the participants are in any debate. They select who to interview and the amount of coverage for each participant. As shall be seen in the discussion of health issues below, participants in the debate may be chosen because they represent the dominant understanding of an issue. Those with the weight of power and authority behind them will be selected to contribute to debates. For example, government ministers rather than unemployed people themselves will discuss the experience of being unemployed. However, the media may also give coverage to participants who may not be authoritative in terms of their knowledge or position in society, but who will be 'colourful' or controversial in their views.

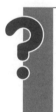

Questions for reflection

What is meant by the term the 'public interest'? Is it possible to reconcile the commercial interests of media outlets with the provision of news and information that is in the 'public interest'?

Constructing meaning

Clearly then, the media are a primary source of information that we use to make sense of our social world. It is not that the media can tell people what to think, but through processes such as agenda setting, the media play an important role in influencing what we deem as important to think about. Further, the way that an issue is framed in the media is critical to the way that we understand the issue. Framing may be described as the presentation of a particular perspective on an issue aimed at eliciting a desired response. There will always be multiple and competing framings of any particular issue. Framing is important because audiences do not have specialised knowledge of all the issues that are raised, and so are dependent upon the perspective or perspectives that are offered. Thus, the media influence people in not only setting the agenda for public discussion, but also in how we may think about current events by controlling the nature and extent of information available about an issue of which the audience has no direct experience. For example, we learn about poverty and HIV-AIDS in African nations, but most of us will never directly experience these.

Further, our experience of distant events is now so immediate and vivid that we feel as though they are part of our own reality. Consider the coverage of the Beaconsfield (Tasmania) miners in May 2006, where 'we' shared the exuberance of the rescue of the two miners. The capacity of the media to bring these events into our daily lives, into our living rooms, means that we are dependent upon them for our 'indirect experience' of the event, and also for their filtering of the information that is available. The filtering process is another way that the media determine what is newsworthy. The parts of the story considered most likely to 'sell' are filtered from other less newsworthy parts of the story.

Through these processes of framing, filtering and providing us with indirect experiences, the media help us to construct meaning. Dominant ideas or constructions are presented using what can be termed 'particular normative constructions'—that is, the presentation of images and stories that accord with the most popular way of understanding an issue. By excluding other possible ways to think about an issue, or by not challenging the dominant ideas or stereotypes that are held, media texts endorse a certain set of social values as inevitable and natural, and reinforce certain beliefs and myths about social identities and cultural norms. These may become entrenched and take on an authority that eludes the pressure of change. These media constructions become considered what 'society' thinks, wants, believes, etc. Petersen (1994: 126) describes this as 'the mobilisation of already existing cultural knowledge'.

The media are therefore important in how we construct meaning about the world around us and how we understand our place in the world. This process of developing self-knowledge applies equally to our knowledge of social events as well as to health and illness issues. 'As the most important source of information, entertainment and increasingly, education, the media are central to our capacity to define ourselves as citizens—not just in terms of electoral choice, but in terms of the self knowledge we are able to distil from the images in news and entertainment' (Schultz, 1994:16).

Question for reflection

How have the media been used to construct meaning around public health issues such as immunisation, childhood obesity and safe sex?

The importance of visuals and language use

We live in a society that privileges visual impact. What we see 'with our own eyes' has a truth value beyond what other people may tell us about an issue, either verbally or in written form. Photographs or live coverage may appear more real and direct than the written word, and the power of visual images is such that we may overlook the fact that images are just as carefully crafted as text. Thus, images in the media can powerfully shape our understanding of issues. Images in the media are powerful because they can act as 'subtext'—conveying unspoken, but intended meanings. For example, a story about differing family forms in Australia accompanied by a visual image of the traditional nuclear family (father, mother and two children) reinforces the dominance of the nuclear family as the preferred model. There is no need to caption such an image as a 'nuclear family'—this meaning accords with a widely understood concept of what it means to be a family in Australia. Such an image can therefore serve to exclude alternative family forms from the consciousness of the reader or viewer, even when the textual message may be about alternative family forms. Such 'juxtapositioning' of image with content may be intentional or unintentional, but the end result may be that the visual image contains a contradictory, but powerful, meaning.

While images are important in the creation of meaning in the media, so too is language. The choice of language shapes meaning through eliciting specific responses or feelings about an issue. 'Selective use of language can trivialise an event or render it important; marginalise some groups, empower others; define an issue as an urgent problem or reduce it to a routine' (Nelkin 1991: 303). 'Lexical style' refers to the choices and variations of words made by journalists. Our meanings and our reactions will change depending on whether media are focusing attention on 'homeless children' or 'street kids', on 'prostitutes' or 'sex workers', in the case of euthanasia on people who 'assist death' versus those who 'murder', whether we see a large gathering as a 'mob' or as a 'crowd'. The significant aspect of language in these examples is that the meaning making is used to attribute a moral judgment about types of people or events. Language can powerfully shorthand an explanation and may be used to deny the complexity of the situation.

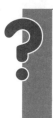

Questions for reflection

Select a current issue in the print media. How important are visual images and lexical style in shaping your understanding of the issue? Can you see alternative ways of conveying information about the issue?

Constructing meaning about health and illness

There is a prevalence of medicine, health and science items in news and current affairs coverage. In fact, such items receive the third-highest coverage after politics and crime stories (Lupton & Chapman, 1994: 95). This is reflective of the contradictory nature of health—on the one hand, it is a social experience with which we can all identify, but on the other, it is a mysterious domain of expert knowledge. This makes it ripe for media interest. In considering our wide social interest in health, we also face contradiction. Health is something that affects us all, but our experience of health is always uncertain, something that cannot be taken for granted. Therefore we have a fascination with stories about health— about people who could be just like us, but have had an experience that 'just as easily could happen to us'. We have strong cultural values around storytelling and health—from handed-down lay understandings about maintaining health or curing illness, to contemporary accounts of health miracles and regimes.

Storytelling is a very poignant way that the media convey both information and entertainment. For example, the story lines in Australian dramas such as *A Country Practice* and *GP* included both illness issues and relationships between the characters. In the past, these programs also focused more on social issues, such as mental illness, alcohol and drug use, and body image. Nowadays, the focus is much more on hospital care and the blood and gore of medical traumas. Health has become an emergency, a life-threatening event. We get drama through *ER*, *House* and *All Saints*, which both entertain and inform us about health and illness. The message that we can always improve ourselves is reinforced through entertainment programs such as *The Biggest Loser*, *Extreme Makeover* and *Turn Back the Body Clock*. There are also hybrid versions of information and entertainment, such as *Is it Good for You?* There is a distinction between news and entertainment media but, as Lupton (1998) demonstrates, the generation of powerful meanings, beliefs and values about health and illness, the health care system and the medical profession occurs just as effectively in the 'entertainment' media as it does in the news.

The media makes the mystery of expert knowledge seemingly accessible. We may never go to medical school, enter an operating theatre or an accident and emergency ward, but we can vicariously experience all of these through media accounts. Our fascination with the processes of health care stems, in part, from a shared bodily existence that is uncertain, as well as a desire to 'see inside' what for many of us is a mysterious domain of expert knowledge. In addition, health and medical work is often deemed to be newsworthy.

We can readily identify differing media discourses about health and illness that promote our interest in viewing health as being about miracles, the bizarre and, overwhelmingly, personal experience. It is through such presentations that media shape our understanding of health and illness in contemporary society and we can identify 'dominant discourses' about health and illness in media coverage relatively easily. The collage of print media headlines provides examples of the ways in which health issues around obesity and lifestyle are conveyed. Consider how meanings are achieved in these headlines as you read through the following ways that discourses about health and illness are presented.

FIGURE 4.1   Headlines

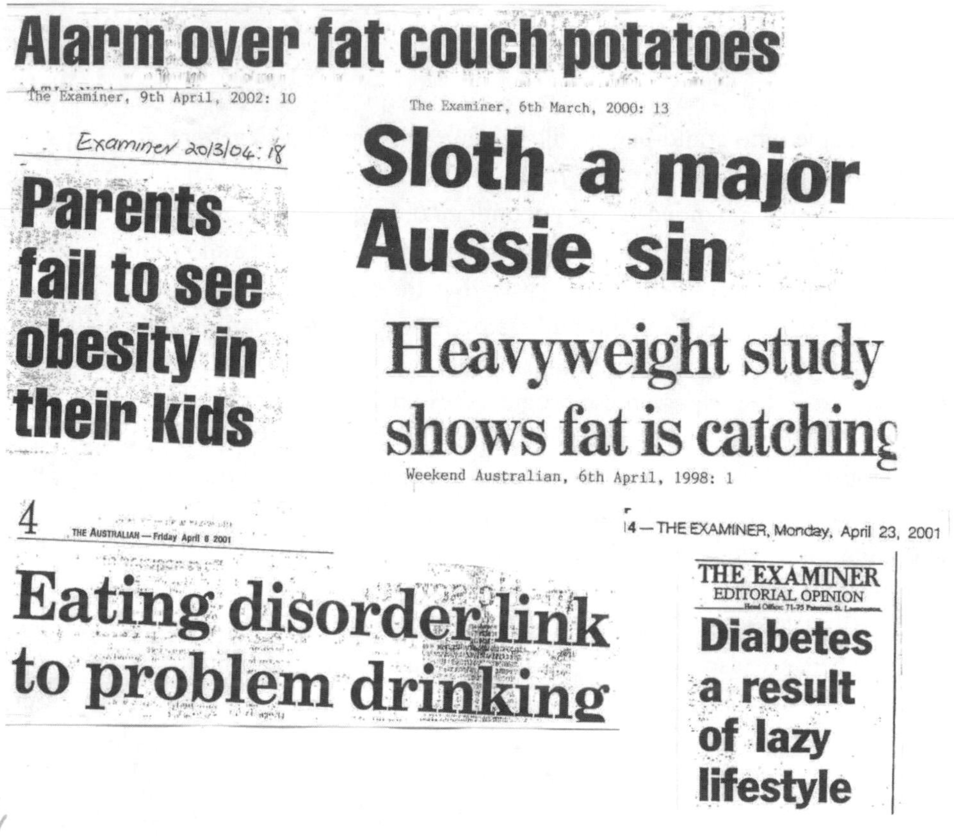

Alarm over fat couch potatoes
The Examiner, 9th April, 2002: 10

Examiner 20/3/04: 18

Parents fail to see obesity in their kids

The Examiner, 6th March, 2000: 13

Sloth a major Aussie sin

Heavyweight study shows fat is catching
Weekend Australian, 6th April, 1998: 1

4   THE AUSTRALIAN — Friday April 6 2001

Eating disorder link to problem drinking

14 — THE EXAMINER, Monday, April 23, 2001

THE EXAMINER
EDITORIAL OPINION

Diabetes a result of lazy lifestyle

Doctors and medicines

Doctors are commonly portrayed as miracle workers, kindly heroes engaged in combat against disease, and patients as a grateful and passive 'our lives in their hands' phenomenon (see Lupton, 1998 for detailed discussion). In the Australian media, the medical profession is portrayed as predominantly white Anglo-Australian men. Medical technology and surgery tend to be accorded a privileged status. The discourses of biomedicine and the uncritical privileging of science are common in the media portrayal of health issues. The moral and social authority of medicine ensures that once an issue is framed as a medical problem, alternative analyses are marginalised. The scientific discourse is a powerful one, and using science as a discourse, health issues tend to be framed as medical problems rather than social issues. This type of portrayal makes it difficult for public health practitioners, who emphasise prevention rather than curative solutions to disease, to have their message heard. For example, Indigenous health issues are routinely presented through a biomedical model that tends to individualise the problem. By locating public explanation of issues within such a framework, complex social causes may be overlooked and not debated, and a victim-blaming response may predominate.

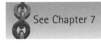

See Chapter 7

Medicalisation

Such portrayal of health issues can be seen as exacerbating trends towards medicalisation. Portrayal of natural events such as pregnancy and childbirth, and social issues such as obesity, drug use and depression as medical problems, reinforces the focus on individuals and 'quick fixes'—for example, the solutions may be found in new technologies, in new drugs, or even in the futuristic promises of genetics.

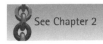

See Chapter 2

Technologies and the 'quick fix'

When mass media cover technologies in health, technologies are viewed as inherently good. This gives rise to the idea of the 'technological imperative'—that is, technological advancement holds the key to solving health problems and that if the technology is available, it should be used. For example, the media coverage of the Human Genome Project (HGP) in particular tends to be as ground-breaking, cutting-edge science in the race to map human genes and, the assumption is, to improve the lot of humankind. However, the HGP is largely decontextualised without consideration for the social and personal consequences of being identified 'at risk' of a 'defective' or 'predisposing' gene. The research is currently very preliminary and the claims made in the media are often extremely premature. While there is some discussion about the social and ethical issues associated with human cloning, the research into genetic links with illness is unquestioned in the media.

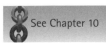

See Chapter 10

Question for reflection

How do media portrayals of stem cell research influence your views of the ethical and moral debates?

Portrayals of health and illness

As well as the construction of dominant discourses in media coverage, there are also dominant portrayals of the experience of health and illness.

Illness as an individual experience

Media coverage tends to individualise the experience of health and illness, locating responsibility in individual behaviour and downplaying the risks posed by wider structural causes and the risk of illness. In this way, illness becomes a metaphor for psychological or moral weakness (Sontag, 1991), a powerful means of placing blame on the ill, or assigning the victims responsibility for becoming ill and getting well. Consider current media coverage of issues such as AIDS, smoking, obesity, anorexia, alcoholism and sexually transmitted infections. In all of these cases, the dominant ideas presented are focused on deviance or individual responsibility, with little acknowledgment of the broader factors that shape exposure to these health risks. Similarly, coverage of legal and illegal drugs depicts socially acceptable drugs such as tobacco, alcohol and prescribed drugs as less dangerous than illicit drugs. Drug problems are related to consumption rather than production, and therefore become the responsibility of the individual.

Illness as a population experience

Illness can also be presented as a 'moral panic'—this is where there is a perceived threat, but where the attention given to it far exceeds the likely risk. In health reporting, moral panics tend to centre on health outbreaks (mad cow disease, food poisoning), emphasising that we are all at risk and focusing on the risky behaviour of individuals (HIV-AIDS). The focus is on sensationalism and raising fear and panic. Such coverage tends to objectify the sufferer and distance the observers or audience from the people and the complex social context in which the issue is located. Early reports on meningococcal suggested that anyone who shared a drink or a smoke could be at risk of contracting the disease. Later reports indicate that it is much more difficult to transmit than originally thought. But still these reports led to anxiety about young child and adolescent behaviour, and to changes in behaviours, particularly in regard to vigilance around children who might intentionally or otherwise share their drink.

People as passive consumers

People are portrayed as 'patients', as passive consumers of medicine, lucky objects of medical miracles or as 'brave fighters in the "war" against illness'. This idea of consumers is particularly pertinent in the coverage of cancer. The importance of this type of coverage is that there we learn about the 'expected response' to devastating and frightening illnesses. Seale (2002) talks about the valorisation of 'ordinary heroes'. He states that 'popular mass media encourages an avoidance of disappointment by overloading media health representations with the spectacle of ordinary people displaying exceptional powers when threatened by illness' (Seale, 2002: 166). In their coverage of the Australian court case of Nadia Maffei, a woman who unsuccessfully sought compensation for wrongful diagnosis of breast cancer, the media portrayed her as a 'saint', 'mother', a 'victim fighting a courageous battle against the odds' and 'a heroine to women across the country'. However, the idea of ordinary sufferers being exceptional denies that there are other ways to experience illness. As Stacey says:

> What of the others? What of those who declined rapidly, who cried with fear and terror in the face of death, who live haunted by the threat of cancer returning or for whom there is no hope? What of those who do not smile bravely? In the success–failure binaries of hero narratives these people can only be seen as failures. (in Shiel, 1999)

People as responsible citizens

The media are important in shaping ideas about what is considered to be the 'normal healthy body'. Ideas about the 'ideal body' focus on the body as a site for body care and maintenance. It is important to remember that the 'ideal body' is historically and socially constructed—that is, what is considered ideal changes over time and according to the different cultural values in society. Our society idealises youth, beauty and slimness. Contemporary lifestyle magazines and lifestyle shows present the consumption of products as a way of achieving these ideals (e.g. gym membership, cosmetic surgery, cosmetics, diet products). Petersen (1994: 133) explains that 'the desires for health, longevity, sexual attractiveness, youth, beauty, and so on, are exploited by the media and distorted in the process of transforming the objects of desire into marketable goods and service'. More important is the idea of the 'rational subject'. Through the portrayal of ideas about the body, media coverage conveys the idea that one's ability to take care of one's own body has become an important marker in contemporary society; evidence of failure to care for one's self is indicative of a flawed and irrational individual. For example, the media coverage of obesity suggests that people become obese because they don't take care of themselves, they eat the wrong food (predominantly fast food) and don't get enough exercise, and that you can't be overweight and healthy. The health problem of obesity is individualised and obese people are viewed as irresponsible for placing their health-risk burdens on the rest of society.

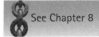
See Chapter 8

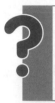

Question for reflection

Which of the discourses listed above do you think is most emphasised in contemporary stories about health and illness?

Information consumption and production: the case of the Internet

Access to knowledge using the Internet has undeniably shaped ideas about health and illness. By using Internet resources, people can be both consumers and producers of health information. The Internet provides an environment in which the users decide what information they are delivered. The range of information that is available has led some commentators to worry about people getting wrong information, while others argue that it can increasingly assist people in managing their health. Search engines don't discriminate—this can challenge the dominance of medical expertise because it challenges the hierarchical models of information provision with which we are most familiar (Hardey, 1999).

The growth of the Internet is illustrative of the rise of the 'information society'. We live in an 'informational environment', where there is an imperative to seek out information about a range of issues, including health. Access to information may be an imperative, but there will be clear social patterning in the production of, and access to, information and the application of knowledge. Giddens (1991) claims that we are increasingly required to be reflexive consumers. Life plans and strategies must be constantly negotiated. This requires sorting through a potentially confusing mass of competing, and possibly contradictory, information. Use of the Internet to gain alternative sources of information may be seen as applying agency and reflexivity in contemporary society where individuals are concerned with gaining control, reducing anxiety and seeking reassurance. The extent to which increased information represents a shift in the capacity of individuals to make choices about health and health care, or functions to reposition consumers and medical professionals, is uncertain. What is certain is that the Internet is a source of information about health worries, concerns or health maintenance. Kivits (2004) claims that the 'informed patient is seeking everyday health information, one reason for which is as a response to poor doctor–patient communication'. Thus the Internet may be used to supplement information provided in a health encounter.

The Internet is a place where information about health issues is shared, expertise built and advice given. The varying ways in which the Internet can convey meanings about health can be illustrated in the multidimensional uses of the information contained. Hardey's (2002) research on the personal websites of chronic illness sufferers is illustrative of the divergent ways in which the experience of illness can be presented by individuals without reliance on third parties (journalists, media organisations) to convey their accounts. Gillett's (2004) research on Internet sites relating to HIV-AIDS found that sites were constructed to provide autobiographical accounts as an alternative source of expertise, self-promotion of cures and products. He also noted that a small minority of sites had dissent as their organising theme. In narratives of health and illness, lay people become experts. It is here that there may be a challenge to expertise, because it is through the sharing of information that professional and experiential knowledge is juxtaposed. Hardey (2002) argues that as patients become experts in their illness, the Internet becomes a vehicle for them not only to share their experience, but it may also be used to sell their expertise.

 See Chapter 3

The multidimensional nature of the Internet is thus an important site for health information production and consumption. Unlike other media forms, the Internet can enable a wide range of individuals to become producers of knowledge, in addition to being knowledge consumers. In an informational society, health professionals must recognise the challenges as well as the opportunities that are presented by increasing access to information.

Questions for reflection

Do you use the Internet as a source of health knowledge? Does the information you receive help you to make decisions about your health?

Exercise: Analysing the media

How can we use our understanding of media to analyse the ways in which the media shape our ideas about health and illness? To ascertain the dominant ideas, beliefs, practices and assumptions portrayed in the text, it is important to consider the following four questions:

1   *What is the overall structure of the text?* Here we need to consider where the story is placed in terms of the overall product. For example, with print media, we need to consider the page where the item is located, the headline, the message in the lead paragraph and whether other ideas and sources are juxtaposed with the item under analysis. We may examine the extent to which an issue is personalised—that is, the way the story is conveyed through an examination of one's personal experience, which may mean that a more emotive portrayal is conveyed.

2   *How are visual images and language used to persuade audiences to accept a particular representation of an issue?* We need to focus attention on the type of language—is it sensationalist, does the headline convey a different message to the rest of the article, does the article use stereotypes to convey a message, and which words and phrases are used? How do these words and phrases 'come together' to shape our understanding? Similarly, with visual images, are photographs or cartoons used, and to what effect?

3   *Whose voice is heard?* Does the story rely on authoritative sources that are deemed credible because of their status in society, or because of the use of scientific knowledge (conveyed with graphs and tables)? It is here that we examine whose voices are heard and whose are silent; who is telling the story and who is having their stories told for them.

4   *Whose interests are served by the reproduction of these particular ideas in the texts?* In exploring this final question, our analysis should uncover who benefits by having this story told, and thus how dominant interests may be reproduced through the media coverage.

Select three newspaper items about current health issues. Analyse these news items with reference to the four questions above.

CONCLUSION

The media play a crucial role in providing information about health and illness through a variety of means. These can range from the presentation of news about health and illness in print and electronic media; entertainment; to the consumption and production of information on the Internet. Analysing media text enables us to critically examine how dominant ideas and values are constructed and presented.

REVIEW QUESTIONS

1   How does mass media contribute to our understanding of the social world?

2   Who has vested interests in the media in contemporary Australia? What are the consequences of this?

3   Why is it important for nurses to understand how meaning is constructed in the media?

KEY TERMS

Agenda setting	Lexical style
Democracy	Mass media
Dominant discourse	Moral panic
Filtering	Network society
Framing	Public interest
Global village	Reflexive consumer
Information society	Subtext
Internet	Visual impact
Juxtaposition	

FURTHER READING

Barr, T. 2000, *Newsmedia.com.au: The Changing Face of Australia's Media and Communications*, St Leonards, Allen & Unwin.

Castells, M. 2002, 'The Internet and the network society: series editor's preface', in Wellman, B. and Haythornthwaite, C. (eds), *The Internet in Everyday Life*, Oxford, Blackwell, pp. xxix–xxxi.

Giddens, A. 1991, *Modernity and Self-identity: Self and Society in the Late Modern Age*, Cambridge, Polity.

Holmes, D., Hughes, K.P. and Julian, R. 2003, *Australian Society: A Changing Society*, Frenchs Forest, Pearson Education.

Kivits, J. 2004, 'Researching the informed patient: the case of online health information seekers', *Information, Communication & Society*, 7, pp. 510–30.

Lupton, D. 1998, 'Medicine and health care in the popular media', in Petersen, A.R. and Waddell, C. (eds), *Health Matters: Sociology of Health and Illness*, St Leonards, Allen & Unwin, pp. 194–207.

O'Shaughnessy, M. and Stadler, J. 2005, *Media and Society: An Introduction*, South Melbourne, Oxford University Press.

Petersen, A.R. 1994, *In a Critical Condition: Health and Power Relations in Australia*, St Leonards, Allen & Unwin.

Seale, C. 2002, *Media and Health*, London, Sage Publications.

Part 2

Social Structure and Health

In Part 2 of this book we examine the relationship between social structure and health to demonstrate how a sociological approach shifts the focus from sick individuals to wider social issues. We achieve this by analysing patterns of health and illness to discover how groups in society experience health and illness differently and how these experiences are not just different, they are unequal. This part examines the impact of social structure and further, it highlights how some social groups are more vulnerable than others to the effects of social structure.

The first chapter in this part, 'Health and Illness Patterns in Australia', explains how health and illness are socially produced and distributed. Social class, gender and ethnicity are examined in depth and the health impacts of social structure are illustrated through case studies of occupational health, domestic violence and refugee mental health. A more nuanced understanding of the influence of social structure is presented in Chapter 6, 'The Health Effects of Marginalisation and Exclusion'. In this chapter, we argue that being excluded from, or marginalised in, mainstream society carries with it particular risks to health that are depicted in case studies of ageing, rurality, poverty and sexuality. The final chapter in this part, 'The Health of Aboriginal and Torres Strait Islander Peoples', extends our analysis of social structure and the social processes of marginalisation and exclusion. We argue that Aboriginal and Torres Strait Islander people's health disadvantage needs to be considered in the broader context of social disadvantage, inequality and exclusion, political marginalisation and the historical currents of colonialism.

Chapter 5

Health and Illness Patterns in Australia

Introduction

Julia had always thought of illness as an individual experience. Even though she was aware that some groups of people seemed to be sicker than others, she struggled to use her sociological imagination—that is, to see private troubles as public issues—to grasp the social distribution of health and illness. Yesterday, Julia watched a television program about the health problems for people living in an outer suburb of the capital city. While she knows that not all people living there are predisposed to getting sick, it became evident that problems like asthma and other respiratory diseases seemed to occur in a patterned, rather than disordered way. It wasn't the well-educated professional people who were shown on the program, but largely people who lived in public housing.

Julia wondered whether or not the same sort of patterns of health and illness occurred in other suburbs. By applying her sociological lens, Julia questioned whether men were prone to illness less or more than women, if older people were sicker than younger people, if people from particular ethnic backgrounds were susceptible to illness more than others, and if people living in certain areas of a city had different health issues than those who lived in the country. There seemed to be an array of possibilities that helped Julia to speculate that people's experiences of health and illness are structured by social factors, rather than being experienced only as individual troubles.

Despite widespread improvement in the health of Australians during the twentieth century, there is considerable evidence of health inequalities between different population groups, which suggests that these health gains have not been equally shared and that these inequalities have social origins. An understanding of patterns of inequality in health and illness helps to explore why different groups in society experience unequal health status and why some groups experience similar problems. In focusing attention on the social dimensions of such patterns, we gain a different perspective on these issues to that obtained from individual or biological explanations.

This chapter explores the ways in which health and illness are socially distributed in Australian society. Following an examination of the nature of the social distribution, we turn our attention to explaining some of the key variables that shape these patterns. By introducing the idea of social structure, we examine how social class, gender and ethnicity shape the experience of health and illness. We conclude that the concept of social structure, and its influence on social positioning, helps to explain the patterns of health and illness that are observed.

Objectives

At the conclusion of this chapter you should be able to:

- understand and apply the concept of social structure to the study of health and illness
- explain how health and illness are socially produced and distributed
- critically examine the health effects of social class, gender and ethnicity in contemporary Australian society.

Social patterns of health and illness

Patterns of health and illness are usually described in terms of their incidence and prevalence. These are epidemiological terms. Incidence refers to the number of new cases of an illness during a specified period. The incidence rate is the number of new cases divided by the number of people at risk of the disease. Prevalence refers to the total number of cases of a disease in the population, rather than simply the number of new cases (Mulhall, 1996). Information about the incidence and prevalence of illness in the community is based upon studies that use various research methods to survey and collect data across the population and population groups. Studying the raw data, examining the relationships between a range of variables and drawing on sociological theories to develop the analysis enables sociologists (and others) to identify the patterns of health and illness.

See Chapter 3

Taking a sociological approach to health and illness reveals that health problems, while they are obviously experienced at an individual and physical level, can be understood as social issues. Rather than focusing on the individual person, we look at the relationships between, and the influence of, social meanings and practices relating to age, gender, ethnicity, culture, employment status, income level, education opportunities, living environment and the associated social power relations to explain, not only what patterns of health and illness exist, but also why they exist.

The social distribution of health and illness is clearly evident when we look at the example of life expectancy, which is used as a measure of population health. In Australia, there has been a significant increase in life expectancy as a result of decreases in mortality (death) and morbidity (sickness) from infectious diseases and cardiovascular disease; however, life expectancy is not shared uniformly across population groups. The average life expectancy at birth in 2002–04 for males was 78.1 years and 83.0 years for females; however, life expectancy for Aboriginal and Torres Strait Islander peoples is about 20 years less. Further, people who are in the lowest socio-economic group can expect to live about three years less on average than their wealthy counterparts (Australian Institute of Health and Welfare, 2006: 4). Other examples of differences across population groups are provided in Box 5.1 (see p 80).

Social structure

Sociologists refer to social structure to explain the ways in which our society is organised. Think about the social interactions that you have each day—with your family, friends, school or university, bank, church, work or shop. Each of these interactions is influenced by the way they are organised—for example, in relation to your social group and where these interactions take place. If you look more

Box 5.1

- Babies born to Aboriginal or Torres Strait Islander mothers are twice as likely to be classified as low birth weight compared to live-born babies of non-Indigenous mothers (Australian Institute of Health and Welfare, 2006).
- Young females living in regional areas in 2001 were 30 per cent more likely to be overweight or obese than those living in major cities (Australian Institute of Health and Welfare, 2006).
- The injury death rate for Aboriginal and Torres Strait Islander peoples is three times as high as for other Australians (Australian Institute of Health and Welfare, 2006).
- Socio-economically disadvantaged groups experience more ill health and are more likely to engage in risky or harmful health-related behaviours (Turrell et al., 2006).
- People aged 25–64 years working in less skilled occupations were more likely to engage in a number of risky or harmful health-related behaviours (Turrell et al., 2006: 177).
- More females (24 per cent) than males (14 per cent) reported using medications for mental health and well-being (Australian Bureau of Statistics, 2006: 9).
- Females were more likely to consult health professionals than males (Australian Bureau of Statistics, 2006: 13).
- Immigrants from culturally and linguistically diverse backgrounds experience a disproportionately higher rate of occupational injury (Lin & Pearse, 1990).

Question for reflection

How can we explain the health differences that are documented in Box 5.1?

closely at these interactions, you may see patterns that emerge—for example, there may be interactions with people of the same age, social class, ethnicity or gender. These are examples of social groups within the social structure. 'The concept social structure expresses the idea that social formations are organised along patterned lines which endure over time and which act as a constraint on those living within them even though those people may not be aware of this' (Van Krieken et al., 2006: 10). The more formal social structures in our society are known as social institutions and they include family, education, religion, health care, government, economy and media. These formal structures significantly influence the formation of social groups and social interactions.

In exploring the social distribution of health and illness, we are undertaking a 'structural analysis' of the whole of society, a macro perspective. Such an approach seeks to 'understand and explain behaviour through consideration of the significance of social institutions and membership of social groups' (Najman & Western, 2000: 5). A structural analysis considers the wider social and environmental conditions of a person's life. This type of approach sees the organisation of society as a key determinant of human behaviour; therefore, in order for behaviour to change, social change is essential (Khan, 2000).

Building on a structural perspective, we also examine the way that factors such as gender, age, social class, ethnicity and culture are socially constructed. By this we mean that these factors are socially created—that is, they emerge from our social relationships and structures. For example, social class is created from a mix of social factors such as income, education and occupation that locate us within the social structure. These factors are also socially defined and in this way they are historically and culturally determined. They are reinforced and perpetuated through the various social practices that accompany them. Social constructionists argue that these factors are not innate—for example, that gender is socially ascribed in terms of masculinity and femininity rather than the biologically determined characteristics of male and female. Importantly, viewing these factors in this way asserts that they are not fixed, unchanging social realities or structures. As a result, we can challenge their existence and begin to see things differently.

Applying a social constructionist viewpoint to the experience of others heightens our awareness of the fact that people experience life differently, that people in different social locations have had different life experiences and this leads to different ways of knowing reality. This perspective also draws attention to the fact that these experiences are not only different, but they are also unequal.

In the same way that we experience social life differently, we also experience health and illness differently. These differential experiences lead us to explore the notion of inequality as it applies to health and illness. The distribution of health and illness, when described in terms of measurable variations in health status between social groups, is referred to as health inequality (Keleher & Murphy, 2004: 5). In recent times, health inequalities have received a great deal of research and attention, particularly in the developed world, where overall health status has improved but is not equally shared among the various population groups. The concept of life chances is useful in understanding the social distribution of health and illness. Life chances 'refers to the chances individuals and groups have of obtaining those things defined as desirable in their society, such as wealth, power and prestige' (Van Krieken et al., 2006: 214), leading to the argument that 'life chances are not equal for everyone, and the quality of life at any age, including experience of good health and well-being, is dependent upon one's access to resources' (Petersen, 1994:1). These resources include ownership of property; satisfying and well-paid employment; adequate income support for those without paid employment; a well-balanced diet; education opportunities; housing; social support; and access to participation in decision making (Petersen, 1994: 1).

The following discussion will provide you with an overview of the social distribution of health and illness in Australia with regard to the three key structures of class, gender and ethnicity. In following chapters, we will extend our discussion by focusing on groups that are marginalised or excluded in Australian society and the health of Aboriginal peoples in Australia.

See Chapters 6 and 7

Social class

Social class refers to patterns of structured inequality based primarily on economic stratification. Economic factors included in defining social class comprise ownership of material goods and money; however, non-economic factors such as education, qualifications and skills are also important. While the theorist Karl Marx saw ownership of property and wealth (capital) as the key determinant of social class, his view of class was extended by Max Weber, who included skills, status (or social honour) and political affiliation or group membership (party) as important. Pierre Bourdieu broadened Marx's view of capital to include all the resources that are available to a person, as indicative of their class position. As well as economic capital, these include 'cultural capital' (cultural knowledge, education), social capital (social connections) and symbolic capital (respect, reputation) (Van Krieken et al., 2006). Sometimes the term socio-economic status is used to refer to a combined measure of these factors (income, education, occupation) when determining social class location.

The existence of health inequalities related to social class or socio-economic status has been substantiated in all countries that collect the data. The Australian Institute of Health and Welfare (2006) reported that 'the health burden in the Australian population attributable to socio-economic disadvantage is large; and much of this burden is potentially avoidable'. The most significant predictor of health status is income. In Australia, low family income is generally linked to poorer health. For example, adults aged 25–64 years in low-income families reported much worse self-perceived health status than adults in higher income families (Department of Health and Aged Care, 1999). In addition, people with lower incomes are less likely to engage in preventative health measures such as sun protection and using screening services, and are more likely to have lifestyle risk factors such as smoking, overweight and lack of exercise (Turrell et al., 2006). There is also evidence that indicates patterns of health service usage also vary by income. For example, people in low income families report substantially higher usage of health services, including hospital admissions and doctor visits (Australian Institute of Health and Welfare, 2006). The impact of material disadvantage is evidenced through differential exposure to societal resources such as housing, safe home and community environments and parental supervision. For example, one of the risk factor indicators in the National Health Survey is food insecurity, or instances where people ran out of food and could not afford to buy more (Australian Bureau of Statistics, 2006).

A person's level of educational attainment is important because of the potential to gain future employment and derive an income. Research by Turrell et al. (2006) supports the link between educational attainment and health status. They found that when compared with their counterparts with a bachelor degree or higher, males and females aged 25–64 years with no post-school qualifications:

- rated their own health more poorly
- reported a higher incidence of illness
- were more likely to engage in risky health-related behaviours such as smoking and insufficient physical activity
- were more likely to report risk factors such as hypertension and obesity.

Occupation also has an indirect influence on health through its association with income and educational attainment, whereby people working in blue-collar or white-collar occupations, with lower status or skill levels, experience greater morbidity and health service use than people working as managers, professionals or administrators (Turrell et al., 2006).

Explanations for health inequalities related to social class

In seeking to explain the causes of health inequalities between social classes, Blane (1985) points to the following four possible explanations:

- **Artefact:** The claimed relationship between social class and health is artificial because it relates to the way that we measure social class rather than to an actual health difference between the classes.
- **Natural or social selection:** Health inequalities are due to biological inferiority, thus healthy people are upwardly mobile.
- **Cultural or behavioural:** Health is influenced by social class behaviours or cultures with ill health being a product of unhealthy behaviour.

- **Materialist:** Health is a result of structural inequality. Illness is influenced by poor living and working conditions, poverty, discrimination, lack of educational and employment opportunities, nutrition, housing, income and savings.

Wilkinson et al. (1998) have added another possible explanation:

- **Psychosocial/social capital:** Income inequality produces psycho-social stressors, such as shame, that negatively impact on health. A social gradient or continuum of health inequality exists whereby health gradually declines as you move down the hierarchy. This explanation has also been linked with theories about social capital because communities with greater income inequalities have been found to lack social organisation, trust and cohesion (Forbes & Wainwright, 2001)

Question for reflection

Which of the explanations for the effect of social class on health do you find most convincing?

The impact of social class: work and health

It is estimated that each year in Australia there at least 2900 work-related deaths. Around 430 compensated fatalities each year are traumatic workplace deaths—the remainder are attributable to work-related diseases (Driscoll & Mayhew, 1999). Type of occupation has a direct influence on health through exposure to workplace hazards, with the highest numbers and rates of injury observed in occupations that are likely to involve physical labour. Mining recorded the highest incidence of work-related injury or illness, with 8.8 per cent of employed persons experiencing a work-related injury or illness, followed by transport and storage (7.8 per cent) and construction (6.9 per cent). Agriculture, forestry, fishing and manufacturing also recorded high incidences of work-related injury or illness. In contrast, finance and insurance (2.2 per cent) and property and business services (2.4 per cent) both recorded a low incidence of work-related injury or illness (Australian Bureau of Statistics, 2000).

Individual action is often the focus for explaining occupational injury issues, with explanations around carelessness, malingering or even age being considered. However, the large number of workers whose health is affected points to the need to see this as a public issue rather than as a private trouble. A sociological analysis focuses attention on the type of work involved (the prestige) and the organisation of work—exploring in particular the practices that may lead workers in some occupations to be exposed to greater hazards. Quinlan and Bohle (1991) point to the range of factors associated with the organisation of work that may increase the risk of occupational injury or disease. These include incentive payment systems, excessive production pressures, shiftwork, compressed or irregular working hours, deskilled and repetitive work, and subcontracting. The experience of working in a globalised society is now often characterised by lower job security, higher rates of contract or casualisation of work, and increased performance pressure, all of which carry attendant risks, either of accident, injury or longer-term health problems. A sociological analysis highlights the tension between profits and worker safety, and the power of workers to enforce safe working conditions. Additionally, as gatekeepers to the 'sick role' and to compensation, health professionals play an important role in occupational health and safety issues.

Shiftwork and overtime are work features that dramatically affect health. They are widespread in industries such as transport, communications and health, and where automated machinery is used. While the effects of shiftwork such as sleep deprivation, irritability and deprivation have been linked with more serious conditions, they are more confidently associated with the higher rate of accidents that occur among workers on night shift, afternoon shift and overtime, than those on normal (day) work (e.g. Harrington, 2001).

Occupational illness is also linked with stress. While stress is commonly thought to be associated with executive and high status positions, there is a growing body of literature suggesting that workers in high demand, low control and low social support jobs are at increased risk of occupationally induced stress or diseases such as cardiovascular disease. George and Davis (1998: 296) cite a study of Brisbane bus drivers where the increased demands of the job meant that they worked in an environment conducive to continual experience of stress, with marked symptoms of distress covered by self-medication.

Questions for reflection

How do contemporary work practices place workers at risk? Is there a social class division that is apparent in exposure to risk due to occupation?

Gender

Health experiences and health outcomes for men and women are different. Men, at all ages, have higher mortality rates than women. However, while women can expect to live longer than men, they have greater contact with the medical system.

There is an important distinction between sex and gender—sex refers to the biologically determined features of being male or female, whereas gender refers to the cultural and social definitions ascribed to being male or female. Thus, gender refers to the way that biological differences are interpreted and translated into the social expectations and experiences in everyday life. Gender constructions are not static—our gendered identities are produced, performed and 'reproduced' in interactions with others.

Gender is contentious and often confronting because it also refers to the unequal distribution of power between men and women. Thus, it is claimed that we live in a patriarchal society—one in which women's interests are subordinated to the interests of men. Power in such a society takes many forms, from the sexual division of labour and the social organisation of families, to the internalised norms of femininity and masculinity by which we live. The social meanings given to biological sex differences are said to be 'ideological'. An ideology is a system of ideas, beliefs and values, which offers a coherent view. Ideologies are not necessarily either true or false. They are perspectives on the world that favour the interests of certain groups.

Another reason that taking a gendered perspective in health is contentious is because such an analysis is considered to privilege one group, generally women, over another, men. A concern with women's health is evident within the feminist movements of the 1960s because health was considered to be an important factor in gender inequality, and was included in broader demands for equality in a patriarchal society. It is only in recent years that the impact of social structure, in particular masculinity, has been analysed as detrimental to men's health. We argue that exploring gender and health is not a 'me too' battle of the sexes—rather we need to critically examine the evidence that relates health to gender, and then put forward possible explanations. These explanations are not about inattention to one sex, but rather relate to different gendered experiences that emphasise the ways in which the social experience of being a man or woman in our society shapes these differences.

The National Health Survey is a five-year self-report survey that asks a cross-section of the Australian population about their health status, health actions and use of health services in the two-week period preceding the survey. A selection of the results from the 2004/2005 National Health Survey points to the different health experiences of men and women.

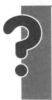

Question for reflection

What are the possible explanations for the differences between men and women in the listed conditions, events and consultations shown in Box 5.2?

Box 5.2

Selected statistics from the National Health Survey (Australian Bureau of Statistics, 2006), used with permission from the ABS

	Males (000)	Females (000)
Long-term conditions:		
Alcohol and drug problems	115.9	45.4
Mood (affective) problems	415.3	637.3
Anxiety-related problems	384.1	583.8
Migraine	375.4	919.4
Angina	126.4	88.0
Varicose veins	134.9	374.5
Hernia	273.2	139.9
Injury events		
Vehicle accident	30.9	10.2
Low fall	349.4	420.9
Attacked by another person	40.6	28.9
Smoker status		
Current smoker (daily)	1782.5	1397.6
Never smoked	2843.1	4144.8
Health service use		
Hospital inpatient	77.8	73.2
Visited casualty/emergency	90.2	87.4
Outpatients	165.0	199.4
Day clinic	212.3	276.2
Consulted GP or specialist	1945.2	2542.5
Consultation with chemist	272.7	492.8
Consultation with naturopath	35.6	97.9
Consultation with nurse	98.2	145.6
Consultation with psychologist	57.7	55.7

Women's health

The assumption of 'sickness being feminine' gives rise to the explanation that women report more illness because it is more acceptable to do so, they have greater awareness of their symptoms, or they have been socialised into greater awareness of possible signs and symptoms, thus more often reporting 'trivial' illness. This explanation, however, tends to simplify the different life experiences, understanding of health and responses to illness that women show, particularly in comparison with men. Men have greater use of hospital services, even though women have greater contact with the health system (largely through the medicalisation of menstruation, reproduction and menopause). Further, there is little evidence of women over-reporting conditions, either long term or trivial, in comparison with men (MacIntyre et al., 1999; Parslow et al., 2004).

There is general agreement that a combination of factors contribute to gender differences in health. While factors such as biology and psychology are acknowledged (Bird & Rieker, 1999; MacIntyre et al., 1999; Zadoroznyj, 2004), the context of social structure is seen as critical to understanding how these factors are given meaning in contemporary society (Denton et al., 2004). Thus, explanations for women's health can be found in considering both the social structures that contribute to health, and medical responses to women's health (Doyal, 1995). Taking into account social changes, including the patterning of work and family responsibilities, it has been suggested that exposure to risk through work and family is fundamentally different for women. The clustering of women in occupations that are likely to be sedentary, low paid, and often repetitious with little job control poses particular risks, particularly musculoskeletal disorders (Strazdins & Bammer, 2004). Further, women predominate in a workforce that is increasingly unstable, comprising a greater number of casual and part-time workers. And while occupation is important in considering health and health risk, what must also be considered is that women continue to be the primary carers for children and informal carers for ill and disabled relatives, at the same time as their participation in the paid labour force is increasing. Strazdins and Bammer (2004) argue that it is the combination of work and family responsibilities that is fundamentally different for women's health.

Sex-stereotyping of women has also contributed to women's experiences of health and, in particular, in their encounters with the institution of medicine. Evidence suggests that clinicians bring stereotypical views of women and men to their clinical decision making. Medical knowledge is not simply objective, value free and devoid of the values underlying the social context in which it is created. One example is the textbooks on obstetrics and gynaecology that contain, and reinforce, sex-stereotyping of women as 'inherently weaker' than men (Koutroulis, 1990). Cardiac disease is another example. Portrayed in both lay and medical circles as a disease of affluence that primarily affects men (Lockyer & Bury, 2002), cardiac disease is not only strongly linked to low rather than high socio-economic status, but is also the number one killer of women. Yet, studies show that women are less likely to receive a diagnosis of cardiac disease when presenting with symptoms (Arber et al., 2006; O'Donnell et al., 2006) and that they are less likely to be referred for investigations, treatment and rehabilitation (Lockyer & Bury, 2002). 'These studies indicate a systematic and troubling difference in physicians' approaches to how male and female patients with essentially the same condition will be treated' (Zadoroznyj, 2004: 144). One consequence of the medical construction of women has been the exclusion of women from scientific trials—thus knowledge construction about women, their health experiences and outcomes has been limited.

Another important explanation for women's health, which locates their experience within the institution of medicine, is the process of medicalisation. Women tend to come into contact with the medical system because normal life events have become medical events—for example, contraception, reproduction and menopause. 'By contrast there are no equivalent, regularly occurring events in men's lives that have been correspondingly medicalised or declared medical problems' (Zadoroznyj, 2004: 139).

Thus, explanations for women's health must take account of two factors—first, their social location as women in a gendered, patriarchal society in which they have less institutional power than men; and second, the way that medicine has constructed knowledge about women in the context of a patriarchal society, where the dominant discourse has been around women's roles in the private sphere of the family, with medical knowledge used to focus attention on reproductive and family functions.

Men's health

Insights into how gender affects men's health have been informed by the way that masculinity is enacted in our society, with some theorists arguing that masculinity exerts greater pressure to conform to societal gendered ideologies than femininity (Courtenay, 2000). While ideologies of masculinity convey the way that men have greater power in society, there is also a gender order that exists within masculinity. Connell (2005) claims that such 'multiple masculinities' are constructed not only as a relation of domination over women, but also in relation to other men, and in conjunction with structures such as social class and ethnicity.

The most dominant form of masculinity is 'hegemonic masculinity'. Hegemony refers to the ideas that are dominant, and that are accepted as dominant by the population, and that provide a public face to these ideas. Thus hegemonic masculinity is dominant over all femininities and other forms of masculinity.

This dominant form of masculinity is the cultural norm that 'valorises and rewards physically aggressive, competitive, task-focused, achievement-oriented masculinity and inferiorises all forms of femininity' (Wearing, 1996: 57).

The gender hierarchy among men involves patterns of domination and subordination. For example, homosexual men are oppressed by overt discrimination, political and cultural exclusion, abuse and physical violence. In this way, gay masculinity is seen as a subordinate masculinity.

While the number of men who vigorously practise the hegemonic pattern might be quite small, the majority of men gain from its hegemony because men in general benefit from the overall subordination of women. Connell (2005) describes this as 'complicit masculinity', which refers to the benefits that are conferred by being in the dominant group, but without the expression of overt power characterised by hegemonic masculinity.

Finally, marginalised masculinities refer to men who have lost most of the benefits of patriarchy due to their subordinate, often marginal, class position or ethnic grouping. The interaction of poverty, unemployment and racism shapes the masculinities of some poor and black men. Themes of hegemonic masculinity are reworked in the context of class deprivation, poverty and racism, and are commonly expressed by what Connell (2005) calls 'protest masculinity'.

Men's health issues are located much more in the broader social (public) arena. Less likely to be the object of the 'medical gaze' than women, their health issues include such things as alcohol, smoking and weight. They have higher causes of death at all ages in such categories as accidents, violence and poisoning, motor vehicle traffic accidents and suicide. While the idea of hegemonic masculinity has been critiqued because it denotes a 'pecking order', with men being dominant over women in a patriarchal society (Macdonald, 2006), hegemonic masculinity, and its associated forms of masculinity, provides a powerful insight into the health risks that men face, particularly when combined with other social structures such as social class and ethnicity.

Ideas about masculinity can inform an understanding of risk exposure. The cultural explanations that facilitate a positive identification of masculinity with risk mean that risky behaviour is not viewed as a medical problem. Risky activities such as dangerous driving, alcohol use, and violent and aggressive behaviour are often explained as simply 'being a lad', and legal sanctions rather than health actions predominate when problems arise (Zadoroznyj, 2004: 132). The sexual division of labour also places men at risk. Not only do men predominate in occupations such as mining, forestry and agriculture where risks are high, but also the performing of appropriate gender identity may be one reason why the risks are deemed acceptable and minimised. Courtenay (2000) also argues that in less overtly risky jobs, such as office or managerial work, the reward structures of prestige, power and pay will negate concerns about health, thus reproducing institutional work structures that reward masculine attributes.

Conformity to dominant constructions of masculinity also affects the likelihood of preventive health actions and compliance with health regimes. For example, Williams' (2000) study of teenagers with asthma and diabetes found that young women were able to incorporate taking medications into their sense of identity, but young men were less able to integrate a treatment plan into their view of what it is to be masculine. A diagnosis of depression also confronts one's sense of self as 'masculine' and research by Emslie et al. (2006) points to how men accommodated the diagnosis in masculine ways, such as re-establishing control, taking responsibility and being 'one of the boys', with a minority of men reflecting on the hegemonic masculinity and attempting to 'do it differently'.

Thus, according to Salstonall (1993) 'doing health is a form of doing gender', requiring analysis of how the different gendered experiences of men and women shape exposure to, and the experience of, health issues. While biology and psychological factors shape health responses, 'a wide range of social processes can create, maintain or exacerbate underlying biological health differences' (Bird & Rieker, 1999: 745).

The impact of gender: domestic violence

One issue that illustrates the effect of gender in contemporary Australian society is domestic violence. While men are more likely to be victims of violence in public (outside the home), women experience much higher levels of violence in private (in the home). This distinction between the public and private domains highlights key differences in the structuring of gendered behaviour and experience. The effect of domestic violence on women is an important cause of presentation to accident and emergency units, but one that has tended to be unrecognised by health workers, or inappropriately treated (Patton, 2003). It is only when we consider a sociological explanation for domestic violence that a full understanding of the effects and possible solutions can be explored. Willis argues that a sociological understanding of issues must include examination of the historical, structural, cultural and critical dimensions of the problem (in Germov, 2005: 21). In historical terms, in patriarchal societies women have been seen as the property of men, with old English law even allowing men to beat women (as long as the instrument was no wider than the diameter of a thumb). Even in contemporary society, marriage ceremonies sometimes still have the 'father' giving away his daughter to her future husband—a legacy of a patriarchal era. At a structural level, women's inferior position in the workforce (even in contemporary societies), and their roles and responsibilities as caregivers mean that they often have less power in relationships. Further, the family and family home have always been seen as private, not public domains—consider expressions about 'my home is my castle' and 'what goes on behind closed doors'. Thus public knowledge and outrage at domestic violence has, until recently, been muted. This, combined with cultural ideals (often obtained through media representations) of 'romance', 'true love' and the privacy of marriage, means that domestic violence shatters these illusions, bringing an element of shame on the women who cannot fulfil the dream. An understanding of these factors means that it becomes possible to understand why women don't leave violent relationships and the pivotal role that support agencies, including health workers, play in making changes to a society that allows violence against women.

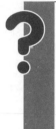

Questions for reflection

What are some commonly held 'myths' about domestic violence. Why do you think they are so powerful in shaping our understanding of this issue? How can a sociological analysis of domestic violence assist health workers in their day-to-day work?

Ethnicity

Australia has one of the most ethnically diverse populations in the world, with approximately one in four Australians born overseas and 52 per cent of population growth from net overseas migration (Australian Bureau of Statistics, 2004a). Approximately half of overseas-born Australians come from non-English speaking countries. There are at least a hundred distinct ethnic groups and this diversity makes generalisation about immigrants difficult. For example, there are significant differences between highly skilled immigrants who come to Australia on a temporary basis to find well-paid employment and those immigrants who are unskilled, from predominantly less developed countries, who experience difficulty getting a job and, when they do, have little security and low wages.

Ethnicity has both sociological and political dimensions. Sociologically, ethnicity refers to a group's collective identity based on shared cultural characteristics, such as language, values, rituals, marriage and kinship patterns, religion and ancestral homeland (Van Krieken et al., 2006: 271). In many cases, ethnicity is constructed around a group identity that emphasises similar characteristics—physical, customary or colonisation or migration experiences. By identifying the similarities of group members, the group distinguishes itself from other groups in society. The political dimension of ethnicity highlights its imprecise and situational nature. For example, in Australia it is used to identify migrants who share a culture that is distinctly non-Anglo-Australian. Thus, a quarter of Australia's population could be affected by this definition when used to denote the non-ethnic majority. Viewed in this way, it becomes evident that ethnicity can be used to determine inclusion or exclusion, and hence the political nature of the concept.

Differentiating between people on the basis of their ethnicity at worst can lead to racism. Racism occurs when actions, attitudes or policies are determined by beliefs about racial characteristics (Abercrombie et al., 2000: 286). Julian (2005: 156) defines racism as 'beliefs and actions used to discriminate against a group of people because of their physical and cultural characteristics'. Racism can be both overt, through targeted acts or expressions against individuals or groups, or it can be covert, less obvious or hidden, and occurring through the systematic exclusion of specific individuals and groups based on their ethnicity.

Health impacts of ethnicity

With the exception of immigrants who enter Australia through the humanitarian or refugee program, almost all immigrants demonstrate good, if not better, health on arrival than the Australian-born population. Their good health lasts for some years after arrival. Their better health status is reflected in longer life expectancy, lower death and hospitalisation rates, and a lower prevalence of some lifestyle-related risk factors. This phenomenon has been explained as the 'healthy migrant effect', with health requirements and eligibility criteria ensuring that generally only those in good health migrate to Australia (AIHW: Singh & de Looper, 2002). The health advantage on arrival is known to become smaller with increasing length of residence in Australia (Young, 1992).Overseas-born persons experienced death rates that were 10–15% lower than for Australian-born persons through the 1990s, but there are instances where mortality rates among overseas-born persons are higher than the Australian-born population (AIHW: Singh & de Looper, 2002). For example, the prevalence of diabetes is high for certain immigrant groups, compared with Australian-born persons, particularly among persons of European, Pacific Islander and Asian origin (Australian Institute of Health and Welfare, 2000).

To understand the health and illness experience of migrants, it is important to understand the socio-historical context of migration in Australia. The changing immigration policies within Australia reflect the power relations between the dominant Anglo-Saxon culture and immigrants. These policies include the White Australia Policy, assimilation, integration, multiculturalism and restricted immigration. In the postwar period, Australia's immigration program emphasised settlement migration to meet economic and demographic needs. This has changed in more recent times towards favouring temporary residents to work in Australia, resulting in significant increases in non-permanent migration (Hugo, 2004). The current Australian migration program includes the following policy components:

refugee and humanitarian movement; family migration; economic migration (including skilled migrants); and special categories. With the changes in migration policy, there have also been changes in the birthplace of overseas immigrants. In the early postwar decades, the United Kingdom, Ireland and countries in Europe were the dominant origins of immigrants. Since the 1960s, there has been an increase in diversity of immigrants from other European countries, but more significantly from Asia, the Pacific, the Middle East and Africa (Hugo, 2004).

The socially constructed nature of health and illness for migrant groups in Australia is evident through the differential experience of migration. Migrating to a new country involves social dislocation, moving from one society to another. Those who migrate experience the transition to a different culture. The migration experience is also affected by the ability to find employment, the stress associated with resettlement, the availability of social support and English-language ability.

For some migrants, their socio-economic status may be lower when they come to Australia. This may be related to the reasons for migration or perhaps non-recognition of overseas qualifications. Many newly arrived migrants have lower incomes and higher levels of unemployment compared to their Australian-born counterparts; however, research has shown that the difference in socio-economic status lessens with the length of time spent in Australia (AIHW: Singh & de Looper, 2002).

Two different, but complementary explanations for varying migrant health experiences and outcomes are culturalist and structuralist explanations.

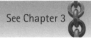
See Chapter 3

A culturalist explanation examines the impact of differing cultural ideas, rituals and practices affecting health experiences. As we saw in Chapter 3, different groups have different understandings of health and illness. Immigrants bring their own particular risk factors, such as diet and cultural practices, which may affect health. Kelaher et al. (2001) report in their study that participants who had changed their diet, or could not obtain their preferred food, were less likely to report being in excellent or very good health. Interactions with health professionals may also be mediated by different understandings of health and illness. Davis and George (1993: 230) claim that medical practitioners dealing with differing cultures are 'least likely to understand the people's outside lives and explanations of their illness. In failing to grasp their patients' explanatory models they are likely to diminish their effectiveness as healers'.

Julian (2005) argues that we cannot consider culturalist explanations in isolation, as there is a tendency towards ethnocentrism in such explanations. Stating that 'ethnicity and class are interrelated' (Julian 2005: 152), she argues that structural explanations must also be sought. For example, location in the occupational hierarchy, and subsequent exposure to work-related injury, is an important factor for migrants. While migrants may come to Australia with above average educational attainment (compared with Australian born), they are less successful in obtaining jobs commensurate with their educational level. Highly educated migrants experience downward occupational mobility or employment due to non-recognition of overseas qualifications, discrimination and devaluation of overseas work experience (Ho, 2006). Similarly, Kelaher et al. (2001) argue that socio-economic issues are major determinants of well-being. The location of migrants in lower status and dangerous jobs not only means that they have less resources for good health, but they have greater exposure to occupational injuries and disease, along with lower rates of rehabilitation from injury (Julian, 2005: 157).

The impact of ethnicity: mental health, refugees and the migration experience

Information from the 1995 National Health Survey found that migrants reported higher incidences of depression and other mental illnesses. Julian (2005) notes some migrant groups, including women, refugees, children and adolescents, and the aged are more at risk of mental illness. While it is thought that social isolation and discrimination pose partial explanations, the lack of acknowledgment of the experience of migration, particularly for refugees, and their subsequent treatment upon arriving in Australia, also constitute major contributors to decreased mental health status. For example, a past history of torture and feelings of insecurity impact on refugees' physical and mental health prior to and after migration. Those who have been granted temporary protection visas still have restricted rights and limited access to social services, including English-language training (Harris & Telfer, 2001).

Asylum seekers are one of the most vulnerable groups. Many of these people have left their country of origin to escape persecution and come to Australia in very difficult circumstances. Whereas other migrants are viewed as making a contribution to the social fabric and economy of Australia, asylum seekers are viewed with suspicion and as a burden (Brotherhood of St Laurence, 2002). They come seeking protection; however, it can take a long time to determine their eligibility to access permanent protection in Australia and in the meantime they may be detained or granted a temporary protection visa. As a result, 'trust is eroded and the refugee feels a great sense of injustice' (Brotherhood of St Laurence, 2002: 4). After their arrival in Australia, they continue to live with fear and uncertainty—fear of being sent back home and the uncertainty of their protection status, and this is likely to contribute to poor mental health.

The fear and uncertainty is amplified for those who are in detention. Sultan and O'Sullivan (2001: 594) describe this as 'detention without trial imposed on people fleeing injustice in a context where no crime has been committed'. The jail-like environment of the detention centre often means that human need is responded to in a way that is punitive and constrains freedom rather than with compassion and dignity (Koutroulis, 2003). Sultan and O'Sullivan (2001) noted a pattern of psychological reactions to detention over time, occurring over four stages, each with increasing levels of distress and psychological disability. The first stage is non-symptomatic, during which the detainee is shocked but remains hopeful that the period of detention will be short. The next stage is the primary depressive stage and follows formal notification that the application for asylum has been rejected and the realisation that there is the risk of forcible repatriation and an extended length of detention. Sultan and O'Sullivan (2001) describe the symptoms in this stage as consistent with a major depressive disorder. The reactions are variable but usually include forms of revolt. The third stage is the secondary depressive stage and usually follows rejection of the application by the Refugee Review Tribunal and results in a depressive illness and a focus on issues of 'self-preservation and survival and an overwhelming feeling of impending doom' (Sultan & O'Sullivan, 2001: 595). The final stage is the tertiary depressive stage, in which the detainee's mental state is characterised by hopelessness, fear, suspicion, rage and resentment. Self-harm during this stage is common.

Children seeking asylum are particularly vulnerable during the process of migration and upon arrival in Australia and their subsequent detention. There are international agreements in place to provide protection for these children, and there is an argument that the existence of a process that 'detains' children contravenes these agreements. A growing body of research has found that the incidence of mental health and psychiatric problems for children is greater for those in detention, even when compared to other asylum seekers with similar pre-migration exposure. Minas and Sawyer (2002: 404) report that 'there is remarkable unanimity of medical opinion: prolonged detention *is* causing harm to the mental health and development of children and adolescents'. The risk is even greater for children who are unaccompanied by a parent or family member. Research indicates that parents can provide some measure of security and stability for children in detention; however, their ability to mediate the impact of detention effectively decreases with the length of time in detention (Sultan & O'Sullivan, 2001).

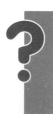

Questions for reflection

What is most important in explaining migrants and health—structural or cultural explanations? What roles can health workers play in the current system where unauthorised entrants to Australia experience detention? What role conflicts are likely to occur for health workers?

CONCLUSION

This chapter has highlighted the inequalities that exist in health status and health outcomes when we consider the impact of the social structures of social class, gender and ethnicity. It is argued that health workers need an understanding of social structure and health, and in particular, how 'the vulnerable and most disadvantaged people of any society are affected by exposure to adverse determinants' (Keleher & Murphy, 2004: 5). Social inequalities mean that health workers work with the vulnerable and the marginalised, as these are the people who experience higher rates of illness events and longer-term morbidity. Khan argues that health workers should take account of socio-economic and cultural factors in day-to-day practice. In fact, ignoring these factors inhibits the capacity to make sound interventions for health. An understanding of the local context is also important in intervening to address health problems (Khan, 2000: 80–1). A structural approach to inequalities in health suggests that a key determinant in improving health outcomes is access to educational opportunities, opportunities for satisfying paid employment, affordable housing, transport and local infrastructure.

REVIEW QUESTIONS

1   How does social structure affect health experiences and health outcomes?
2   Which structural variable impacts most on the health of affected groups?
3   How can health workers take social structure and health into account in their practice?

KEY TERMS

Epidemiology	Mortality
Ethnicity	Prevalence
Gender	Social class
Incidence/incidence rate	Social construction
Life chances	Social inequality
Life expectancy	Social structure
Morbidity	

FURTHER READING

Australian Institute of Health and Welfare 2006, *Australia's Health 2006: The Tenth Biennial Health Report of the Australian Institute of Health and Welfare*, Canberra, Australian Institute of Health and Welfare.

Brotherhood of St Laurence 2002, 'Seeking asylum: living with fear, uncertainty and exclusion', *Changing Pressures*, Bulletin no. 11.

Connell, R.W. 2005, *Masculinities* (2nd edn), Crows Nest, Allen & Unwin.

Doyal, L. 1995, *What Makes Women Sick: Gender and the Political Economy of Health*, Houndmills, Macmillan.

Julian, R. 2005, 'Ethnicity, health, and multiculturalism', in J. Germov (ed.), *Second Opinion: An Introduction to Health Sociology* (3rd edn), South Melbourne, Oxford University Press, pp. 149–67.

Keleher, H. and Murphy, B. (eds) 2004, *Understanding Health: A Determinants Approach*, South Melbourne, Oxford University Press.

Koutroulis, G. 2003, 'Detained asylum seekers, health care and questions of human(e)ness', *Australian and New Zealand Journal of Public Health*, 27, 4, pp. 381–4.

Patton, S. 2003, *Pathways: How Women Leave Violent Men*, Hobart, Women Tasmania, Department of Premier and Cabinet.

Quinlan, M. and Bohle, P. 1991, *Managing Occupational Health and Safety in Australia: A Multidisciplinary Approach*, Crows Nest, Macmillan.

Turrell, G., Stanley, L., de Looper, M. and Oldenburg, B. 2006, 'Health inequalities in Australia: morbidity, health behaviours, risk factors and health service use.' Health Inequalities Monitoring Series No. 2. AIHW cat. no. PHE 72, Canberra, Queensland Institute of Technology and the Australian Institute of Health and Welfare.

Zadoroznyj, M. 2004, 'Gender and health', in C. Grbich, (ed.), *Health in Australia: Sociological Concepts and Issues* (3rd edn), Frenchs Forest, Pearson Longman.

Chapter 6

The Health Effects of Marginalisation and Exclusion

Introduction

The structures influencing health discussed in the previous chapter demonstrate some of the ways in which health and illness are socially patterned. While social structure is important in understanding patterns of health and illness, we must also examine the complexities that exist within this patterning. This chapter focuses on the social processes associated with social exclusion and marginalisation. We argue that being excluded from, or marginalised in, mainstream society carries with it particular risks to health. Based on the premise that access to social support, inclusion in social networks and participation in decision making are important factors in determining health, this chapter explores how social marginalisation is a health issue. Four diverse examples are presented to illustrate the ways that we can consider the health effects of marginalisation and social exclusion: ageing, rurality, poverty and sexuality. This narrows our focus from the 'big categories' of social structure, such as social class, gender and ethnicity discussed in the previous chapter, to a more in-depth consideration of differential experiences within and across these categories. This knowledge enables all health workers (including nurses) to deepen their awareness of social structure.

Objectives

After reading this chapter, you should be able to:

- understand and apply the concepts of marginalisation and social exclusion
- explain how health and illness are the result of social exclusion and marginalisation for some groups in contemporary Australian society
- apply our understanding of the social structures discussed in Chapter 5 to an in-depth understanding of specific structures and specific population groups
- analyse critically taken-for-granted assumptions about the causes of ill health for marginalised groups.

Social exclusion and marginalisation

When groups of people are not able to participate fully in society, they experience social processes that can be identified as social exclusion and/or social marginalisation. Ideas around social exclusion and marginalisation relate to the pivotal nature of citizenship within our society. The notion of citizenship has conventionally been understood as the broad range of rights that accrue to everyone in a society who is deemed a 'citizen'. This is a 'universal' view of citizenship that is predicated on equality. While on the surface the 'equality' view of citizenship seems justifiable, it may overlook some citizens in society who are unable to exercise their rights fully or who need special assistance in order to do so. For example, Medicare provides universal health insurance for all Australian citizens; however, barriers still exist that affect the capacity of some people to access medical services. This points us to the idea of 'equity' as central to our understanding of the capacity to participate fully in society. Equity relates to ideas about fairness and social justice—in the Australian vernacular, to 'giving everybody a fair go'.

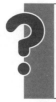

Questions for reflection

Which social groups have difficulty exercising their rights as citizens? What are the reasons for this?

Processes of social exclusion occur when people experience problems such as unemployment, discrimination, low income, poor housing, high crime, ill health and family breakdown. These problems are linked and mutually reinforcing, and in this way many of the causes of social exclusion are also its consequences. Sometimes we refer to people who are socially excluded as people who have 'fallen through the net'. This reflects the process of becoming disconnected from the opportunities available in society. 'Social exclusion refers to a departure from "normal" living standards and implies a power relationship in which some groups exclude others from access to resources' (Van Kriekan et al., 2006: 250). Such a definition locates social exclusion as a social process, rather than a natural or inevitable occurrence in our society.

Sen (2000) argues that social exclusion can be active or passive. Active exclusion is the direct consequence of an intentional policy or practice. For example, active exclusion may relate to workplaces requiring employees to retire when they reach a certain age, thus excluding them from the workplace after that age. Another example is the strict control that is exercised in defining who can, or cannot, become an Australian citizen. Passive exclusion occurs as a result of particular social processes or circumstances, and may be an unintended consequence of a policy or practice. For example, situating a health service away from the public transport route may be seen as passively excluding those potential clients who are reliant on public transport. At a broader level, passive exclusion of people in poverty exists when their poverty and isolation are reinforced and attenuated due to a downturn in the economy (Sen, 2000: 15).

While some commentators see the concept of social exclusion as a useful extension of ideas about inequality, others argue that the definition is not clear-cut, particularly if we do not pay full attention to the range of social processes that may contribute to exclusion from the mainstream of society. Saunders (2003) points out that unravelling the cause and effects of social exclusion is difficult. He uses the example of elderly people who stay at home because they are fearful for their safety. At one level, we may say that they are exercising their choice not to participate in broader society; at another we may blame the behaviour of others (often young people) for causing them to feel fearful. But a broader view would examine public infrastructure issues and economic policies that result in economic uncertainty and unemployment for particular groups. As Saunders (2003: 7) says, 'the aged end up being excluded, but trying to identify what act or acts have excluded them (or led them to exclude themselves) is very difficult'.

The related concept of marginalisation refers to being socially positioned as inferior because of social and cultural perceptions of difference. These perceptions of difference and 'otherness' also result in societal positioning outside mainstream society. The process of marginalisation may not only focus on specific groups, but also on the defining of health issues in particular ways that marginalise alternative points of view. This approach to social positioning is not without its critics. For example, it can be argued that labelling groups as socially excluded or marginalised can mean that we focus our attention on these groups as 'problems' rather than considering the wider social context and processes that create and sustain marginalisation. There is, however, value in identifying how this social positioning and its related discourses can affect one's exposure to, and experience of, health and illness.

Question for reflection

Which groups in our society are most likely to be marginalised on the basis of a perception of 'social inferiority'?

The health effects of social exclusion or marginalisation are inextricably linked with the structural variables we considered in Chapter 5. However, from the perspective of social exclusion or marginalisation, the effects of social class, gender and ethnicity may be exacerbated. Thus location (in terms of social or physical location) and participation (through identity as a full and active citizen) are both contributors to the experience of being socially excluded or marginalised. Hence the broad scope of examples presented in this chapter.

Example one: Older people

If problems such as unemployment, discrimination, low skill levels, low incomes, poor housing, high crime, ill health and family breakdown can result in social exclusion, then older people in our society are certainly more vulnerable than most. While we must acknowledge that there is a biological component to ageing, the conditions under which we experience ageing, and our values and expectations about the ageing process are social and cultural in origin. People aged over 65 years make up 13 per cent of the Australian population (Australian Institute of Health and Welfare, 2006: 215). With the population ageing, and a declining fertility rate, this percentage is projected to increase considerably in the foreseeable future, giving rise to health practitioner, social planning and economic concerns about the 'problem of ageing'. This example will highlight the impact of stereotypes, discrimination and discourses about productivity on the health and well-being of older people.

Stereotypes of any social group can be damaging. Germov (1998: 353) explains that a stereotype is 'an exaggerated, superimposed and generalised portrayal of a group. It involves the adoption of an oversimplified, narrow and standardised image to explain the behaviour or characteristics of individuals and groups'. Stereotypical views of older people include people who have grey hair, receding hairlines and false teeth; are not sexually active; take lots of medications; have poor memory; are bad drivers; and are not physically active. Some commentators claim that our negative stereotyping of age is reflective of our own fear of the process of ageing, and thus we view the aged as 'other' to us:

> Regardless of whether it is white-haired couples striding up mountains, women in cardigans hanging on to zimmer frames, or 'frail old ladies' being looked after with tender loving care, older people are being set apart as people who are 'different from us'. (Bytheway & Johnson, 1998: 256)

A negative stereotypical view of older people can lead to ageism, which is a form of discrimination. 'Ageism "deprives people of power and influence"' (Khun, 1990 cited in Petersen, 1994: 61). Ageism encompasses a broad range of social practices, from institutional polices that abuse and harm people to ageist remarks that dismiss, belittle and insult them. In our society, both the young and old tend to suffer discrimination, most obviously in the area of employment, from which they are more likely to be excluded. However, as Petersen (1994: 61) states 'elderly people are more often victims since, in our society, old age is associated with decay, senility and a reversion to child-like behaviour'. In considering the discourses of ageism, we are responding to the way that age is framed in our society. For example, if old age is framed as a problem, it is responded to in terms of the social problem of an ageing society, such as the problems of supporting more and more people in their old age, and the need for increased health services. The solutions tend to reinforce our attitudes towards the aged as dependent, unable to be productive in society and sick.

A dominant discourse about ageing relates to the idea of productivity and this can also contribute to a range of stereotypes about older people. With an emphasis on the economic productivity in society, the idea of a growing number of people being labelled as unproductive participants contributes to the marginalisation process. Even the notions of 'productive', 'positive' or 'successful' ageing assume that older people have a duty and responsibility to age in a way that is defined by the mainstream as 'good' or 'successful'. And there are changing standards by which people are judged. For example, in recent years, the standing of old people has been markedly lowered since the notion of experience has been discredited. In our modern 'information society', knowledge does not accumulate with years but grows out of date. Definitions of 'successful' ageing come mainly from the field of gerontology (the study of ageing), 'rather than the perspectives of older people themselves' (Nunkoosing & Cook, 2006: 1). Research by Warburton and McLaughlin (2005: 726) refutes the dominant perceptions of the elderly as dependent and unhealthy, instead finding that 'older people, rather than typically being frail and dependent, are instead at the core of the community', contributing in ways that support their families and peers in a manner that is often not valued by experts on productivity.

Questions for reflection

How are dominant discourses about ageing perpetuated in society? Is the discourse of 'productive ageing' necessarily harmful?

The majority of older Australians rate their health as good, while at the same time recognising that health is an important resource for maintaining an active, independent lifestyle that enables social participation and interaction. Most older Australians are neither frail nor in need of long-term care and assistance.

When we examine the popular myth that all old people end up in nursing homes, we find that despite Australia having a relatively high proportion of people in nursing homes, the majority of older people do not live in institutions. However, what can be observed is that as people age, the likelihood of needing long-term care and assistance increases. For example, while 3.8 per cent of people aged 65–84 live in residential care accommodation, this proportion increases to 32.4 per cent for the 85+ population (Gray, 2006: 143). Chronic illnesses account for most of the health issues of the ageing population. These range from the correctable disorders (for example, sight and hearing) to those that cause limitations in living capacity (such as arthritis) and those that in advanced stages require use of medical and hospital services (for example, advanced kidney disease requiring dialysis, or dementia).

When we explore health issues for older Australians, we must examine the extent to which there are the result of biological changes or whether they are exacerbated by the social place of the elderly in our society. Gray (2006) argues that social isolation is an important factor in the illness experience of ageing people. Strazzari (2006) points to the significance of 'social death'—the process whereby elderly people are progressively excluded from the social world. Factors that may impact on social isolation include death of a partner, exclusion from work and lack of resources to maintain social contacts. Keleher (2004a: 316) argues that 'socioeconomic status, lack of transport options, access to health services, and the availability and quality of social supports, are key determinants of the ageing experience'. Further, structural factors are implicated in the health experience of ageing Australians. For example, issues of social isolation may be particularly pertinent for women because the combined effect of women living longer than men and the fact that women are most usually partnered by men older than themselves increases the chance that they will live by themselves while they age. The links between poverty and health are also important: 'Social isolation can increase the risk of health related problems for the aged person, and the poorer the person, the greater risk' (Nunkoosing & Cook, 2006: 1).

Thus, while we cannot deny that biological ageing changes one's physical capacity, and sometimes mental capacity, for many older people the ageing experience is one that is characterised by exclusion and marginalisation, rather than their incapacity to participate.

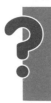

Question for reflection

Why is it important to understand the links between structural position and social exclusion when analysing the health of older Australians?

Example two: Rurality and health

The causes and consequences of social exclusion may also be amplified as a result of geographic location, specifically in rural locations. While there are differing definitions of rural and remote, a commonly accepted definition is that those living in centres and communities with less than 250,000 people can be classified as rural. There are therefore a wide range of geographical environments included in this definition—large regional centres, coastal towns, small inland towns, farms and 'outback' Australia. Using this definition, 34 per cent of Australians can be classified as living in a rural or remote area of Australia (Australian Institute of Health and Welfare, 2006: 239). While rural Australia encapsulates much of the ideology on which our national identity was based, the experience of being physically separated from mainstream Australians, who mostly live in urban, coastal areas, poses a different set of health care issues. In an urban-centric society, such as Australia, those who live outside of urban centres are more likely to experience exclusion from the rights to services and amenities that are taken for granted. The experience of living in rural Australia is qualitatively different to that of their urban counterparts. There are four key areas where we should focus our attention in understanding rural health issues. These are service provision, socio-economic status, the rural environment and rural culture (Gray, 2006).

Rural Australians do not have access to the same level of health care services as their urban counterparts. The changing health care system means greater centralisation of services in regional centres. Regional health services are not only valued for their direct health care contribution, but also for their indirect economic contribution as a source of employment for locals and for bringing people into the communities. Clark et al. (2005) argue that with increased numbers of Australian retirees moving from cities to coastal and rural locations, there will need to be better health services for a population that is more at risk of the diseases associated with ageing (e.g. chronic heart failure). Treatment for long-term or chronic conditions may mean travelling some distance to regional or city centres, exacerbating the effect of social isolation. In some cases, rural location may be a factor in treatment choice. For example, women with breast cancer may choose radical surgery rather than have a prolonged, but less invasive, treatment that would necessitate either travelling long distances over a long period of time or temporarily leaving home. Where services do exist locally, small community settings may make the need for privacy and confidentiality problematic. For example, young people in rural communities seeking assistance, advice or information about sexual health issues are uncomfortable accessing such services if they believe that their need for privacy may be compromised (Hillier & Harrison, 1999).

Socio-economic status is an important indicator of health status. With the exception of mining towns and wine-producing regions (Dixon & Welch, 2000), residents of rural Australia have lower incomes, lower levels of education and less access to employment (particularly skilled employment) (Australian Institute of Health and Welfare, 2006: 239). While housing is cheaper, costs for amenities and food are higher. These factors combine directly and indirectly to impact on health and well-being. For example, low incomes may directly impact on a family's capacity to purchase food or see a dentist. Other factors, such as levels of education and type of employment, may have more indirect influence on breastfeeding, sun protection, use of preventative health care services and engaging in behaviours potentially detrimental to health (Turrell et al., 2006).

Linked with socio-economic status, the nature of the rural environment may predispose residents to differing patterns of illness. Rural employment is more likely to have occupational risks (e.g. farming, forestry, fishing and mining). There are also particular risks associated with travelling in rural areas. Greater distances, hazardous roads and greater likelihood of animals on the road, together with driver issues such as higher speeds and fatigue due to longer driving times, may set up an environment that is potentially more hazardous than urban areas (Australian Institute of Health and Welfare, 2006: 240).

In addition, the stress of living and working in rural areas prone to environmental conditions such as droughts, bushfires and floods also has an effect. Alston's research (2006) points to the impact of gender under such conditions. Men become overworked and socially isolated due to the increased workload. Women face an additional burden—not only are they partners in farming businesses, but women also often seek off-farm employment to assist with family finances, in effect adding an additional dimension to the problems of work/family balance. Women in Alston's (2006: 162) study reported that while health is important, under these circumstances it 'becomes a low priority'.

Although less easy to quantify, it has also been suggested that rural Australians depend on values of independence and stoicism in order to survive, and that this ideology is perpetuated in the way that we view the life of rural Australians. However, such cultural values may also be harmful to health (Alston, 2006). For example, Gray (2006: 88) points to the way that the strong cultural values of stoicism and self-reliance may mean that people in rural areas are less likely to seek help for mental health issues. Combined with a lack of services, this means that it is difficult to ascertain the full extent of mental health issues. The same may be true of other chronic diseases and illnesses that are stigmatised.

Social constructions of masculinity and femininity are important in understanding health in rural areas. It is claimed that rural men's mental health is vulnerable due to changing cultural expectations about gender roles (Wainer &

Chesters, 2000), and that women are more at risk of domestic violence in rural communities. While gender provides a useful framework for understanding the risk of domestic violence, added complexities, such as higher rates of firearm ownership, geographical distances and services such as police that may not respond in a way that fully supports women, are all factors that increase the risks that women face. The issue of reporting domestic violence is particularly sensitive in rural areas. Loxton et al. (2003: 5) found that reluctance to report was exacerbated where women's 'partners knew the police socially, and in one case the woman's partner **was** the local police officer'. Women's sense of belonging in their community may also be threatened if they report domestic violence. Feelings of shame and the experience of stigma, fear of not being believed and becoming the subject of 'gossip' are all barriers to reporting violence (Loxton et al., 2003).

Most commentators agree that there are specific demographic characteristics of rural communities and that on most health indicators, rural Australians experience poorer health. The question about whether this is due to rurality per se, or the social factors that contribute to health, remains contested. For example, deaths from heart failure (Clark et al., 2005) and youth suicide are disproportionately higher in rural areas (Gray, 2006; Dixon & Welch, 2000). There is also evidence that lifestyle risk factors are higher in rural areas. The *Australia's Health 2006* report found higher rates of smoking, hazardous drinking, overweight and inactivity in rural areas (Australian Institute of Health and Welfare, 2006: 239). If we consider the notion of equality as fundamental to citizenship, which is in turn an expression of our rights, then we need to consider whether rural people have the right to expect the same level of health as their urban counterparts; to retire in good health in a town of their choice; and to have access to affordable, accessible and appropriate health care. If so, then we need to question whether rural people are 'getting a fair go' or whether they are socially excluded from mainstream, urban Australia.

Question for reflection

How could you use the information provided above to offer advice to a health worker going to work in a rural area for the first time?

Example three: Poverty, unemployment and homelessness

The concept of social exclusion is most commonly applied to those people who are unable to participate in society because of their economic circumstances

(Keleher, 2004b). Thus, while poverty may be seen as an issue of economic insufficiency, we must also remember that people who are poor or have nowhere to live are excluded in a range of ways. The close link between poverty and social exclusion is seen as important by commentators who argue that this conveys the idea that social exclusion results in involuntary deprivation with pervasive effects (Burstein, 2005). This view of poverty emphasises 'poor living' not just 'depleted wallets' (Sen, 2000: 3). This is what is known as a relational view of poverty—that poverty is more than not having enough resources to survive, it is about an incapacity to achieve what is expected within the broader society. As Sen (2000: 44) argues, 'no concept of poverty can be satisfactory if it does not take adequate note of the disadvantages that arise from being excluded from shared opportunities enjoyed by others'. It is estimated that the number of people living in poverty in Australia is somewhere between 2 and 3.5 million (Mission Australia, 2004). The health effects of poverty are well recognised— lacking basic resources for such things as good housing and nutrition predisposes people to health risks both in the short and longer term. In the following section, we explore the social processes surrounding unemployment and homelessness in an attempt to shift the focus from individual behaviours to social processes.

Unemployment

Employment is seen as a central part of an adult's life, at least until retirement or an inability to work, and as a result there are many social meanings attached to employment in our society. As with the issue of productivity and ageing, the language of employment—our 'working life'—reflects the dominance of this idea. Not only is employment an integral basis of social networking in society and our economic relations, but paid work is also an important source of identity. While these dominant ideas about work are not in themselves destructive or negative, there are implications for those without recognised paid employment. These implications can range from embarrassment, stress, low self-esteem, loss of social status and standing, poverty, stigmatisation and alienation from society, and poor health.

The social problem of unemployment illustrates the concept of passive exclusion as outlined by Sen (2000). For example, passive exclusion is evident in the way that government policies determine who is counted as unemployed, and even when unemployment rates are decreasing, there are many groups seeking work but who are not included in the 'unemployment rate'. These groups are known as the 'hidden unemployed' and include young people who are not in education but who are excluded from applying for Centrelink payments;

discouraged job seekers; partners of employed people who are not working; and people who are in part-time and casual positions, but seeking full-time work. Even when economic times are good, some groups still struggle. The saying 'a rising tide no longer lifts all boats' means that increased job opportunities advantage particular groups in society, and may widen the gap between the haves and the have nots. For example, while increased productivity may create additional jobs, many of these may be in casual and low-paid service sectors, with little job security and additional health risks.

The impacts of unemployment are highlighted further in research conducted with men aged between 40 and 60, living in a small regional centre, in order to find about their experiences of being unemployed or on a disability pension (Cameron et al., 2000). Participants identified the social context of a decreased job market in a rural area, discrimination on the basis of age and gender issues as significant determinants of their health status. All participants identified stress and depression as significant health issues associated with their social status. Issues associated with medical care included being reluctant to see a doctor (but attending frequently), identifying cost as a barrier as well as the inability of doctors to understand their situation on a personal level, or to really assist them on a structural level. These men identified the opportunity to obtain work as the major factor in improving their health. The findings revealed that unemployment, poverty and loss of social identity were identified as the major causes of health problems. Social marginalisation, family tensions and the loss of their identity as the breadwinner (in their family's eyes and also in the broader community) were also linked by the participants to their health issues. Participants clearly identified the compounding disadvantages of their age, disabilities and employment status as locating them at the bottom of the social hierarchy.

While it has not been conclusively demonstrated that unemployment per se causes ill health, there is increasing evidence showing that this is the case. Harmful consequences of unemployment can result from combinations of poverty, stress, social isolation and deterioration of mental health. Compared with people who are working, unemployed people are more likely to experience higher rates of ill health and mortality, a greater prevalence of disability and handicap, more frequent use of medical services and poor or fair health (Mathers & Schofield, 1998). They are at risk of reduced fitness (despite the prevailing view that they must have plenty of time because they are not at work).

Homeless young people

As with unemployment, homelessness poses particular health risks. Young people who are homeless are among the most vulnerable in our society. The number of homeless children 'living on the street' is impossible to measure precisely. However, of the 100,000 people estimated to be homeless in any night, it is claimed that nearly half are aged 25 years or under (Mission Australia, 2005). These comprise those who are 'sleeping rough' (in parks or streets); in temporary or crisis accommodation, in boarding houses with no security of tenure, and marginally housed—living in caravan parks because they are unable to access mainstream housing.

Consider these statements made by homeless young people. Homelessness is like:

A lifestyle which includes insecurity and transiency of shelter.

Absence of shelter

Being on the streets

No place to call home

Living your whole life in public

Homelessness to me was a feeling of death. There is nowhere to go, no-one to see and no-one who cares. (Burdekin, 1989)

Homeless young people have no minimum resources to address health issues. The basic factors for good health, such as adequate nutrition, hygiene, sleep, exercise, low stress and avoidance of substance use, are not available to the homeless young. They have no access to kitchens, bathrooms and laundries. They cannot establish normal sleep patterns. They are constantly at risk of violence and exploitation, and may suffer severe depression as a result of extreme vulnerability, loneliness and hopelessness. They suffer chronic unemployment, lack of financial security and lack of education. This helps to explain the high incidence of drug abuse, violent self-harm and suicide attempts. Poverty can lead to prostitution and sexual exploitation.

While publicity is often given to young people who are choosing to leave home for 'frivolous reasons' or to obtain Centrelink payments, Burdekin states that the situation is usually more complex:

Children and young people leave home because they find family conflict intolerable, are rejected or even evicted, are subject to physical, sexual and/or emotional abuse within the family home, have been ill-served by welfare intervention, need to leave in order to have a reasonable chance of finding work, leave because they were a drain on family finances or because they desire independence. From most evidence it was clear that a complex variety of factors usually precedes the decision to leave. (Burdekin, 1989: 85)

Sexuality
M7 - 113
149.

flection

and long-term health and social consequences
nt and homelessness?

Example .....   lity and social exclusion

A different set of social processes are evident when we consider social
exclusion and taboos around sexuality. Research indicates that people whose
lives exist outside of the heterosexual norm, and normative constructions of
gender, experience considerable stigma from mainstream society. As a result,
they experience marginalisation and social exclusion in multiple and often
reinforcing dimensions, which have a demonstrably negative impact on their
health and well-being. This example describes the processes that contribute to
the marginalisation of gay, lesbian, bisexual, transgender or intersex (GLBTI)
people and the resultant health effects.

While the impact on health of social factors such as age, gender, ethnicity,
culture, employment status, income level, education opportunities and the living
environment are well established, it is notable that sexual orientation and gender
identity receive considerably less attention. Leonard (2002: 4) argues that sexual
orientation and gender identity influence patterns of health and illness specific to
GLBTI people in at least two ways. First, the dominant understandings of sexual
orientation and gender identity serve to discriminate and marginalise GLBTI
people; and second, sexual orientation and gender identity interact with other
social and biological processes to produce patterns of illness specific to each of
these groups (Leonard, 2002: 4).

Two concepts central to our understanding of the processes of discrimination
and marginalisation of GLBTI people are heterosexism and heteronormativity.
Heterosexism is 'the belief that everyone is or should be heterosexual and that
other types of sexuality are unhealthy, unnatural and a threat to society', and it is
used as an umbrella term that includes homophobia and transphobia, which are
essentially fears about alternative sexualities or gender identities (Leonard, 2002:
9). Heterosexism also assumes that sexual identities are fixed and unchangeable.
GLBTI people experience social exclusion as a result of heterosexism and
the reported impact includes violence, isolation, social invisibility and self-
denial, guilt and internalised homophobia or transphobia (Leonard, 2002).
Heteronormativity is a related concept that refers to the generalised view that
heterosexuality is the 'norm' and the heterosexual experience is the only perspective
that is considered (Johnson, 2002). Heteronormative perspectives exclude and

render invisible alternative experiences of sexuality and gender. The assumption of heterosexuality through the processes of heterosexism and heteronormativity operates to demonise and individualise accounts of non-normative sexuality and gender. These processes also deflect attention away from issues that impact on the health and well-being of people outside heteronormativity.

Despite an increasing social acceptance of gay and lesbian people, evidence suggests that accessing health care remains problematic. Consider the data collection on intake forms that ask you to identify as male or female, and as single, married or de facto—how do GLBTI people respond to these questions? Research conducted in Victoria found that 23 per cent of GLBTI people had experienced discrimination in relation to medical care (Victorian Gay and Lesbian Rights Lobby, 2000). Our health services exist in an environment of heteronormativity, and given the lived experience of negative attitudes from health care professionals, the primary concern for many GLBTI people is whether they will experience feelings of acceptance or rejection by the health care agency. This uncertainty impacts on the way that GLBTI people engage with the health care system—for example, late attendance, underscreening and a lack of confidence—and may explain patterns of underutilisation (Pitts et al., 2006).

The health of GLBTI people is poorer than their heterosexual counterparts on a number of different measures. This can be understood when we consider that they have a shared experience of heterosexism, social isolation and invisibility. There are specific patterns of mental, physical and sexual ill health for GLBTI people, as well as common patterns of drug and alcohol use (Leonard, 2002). For example, GLBTI people are more at risk of physical violence and abuse on the basis of their sexuality or gender identity (Victorian Gay and Lesbian Rights Lobby, 2000). This in turn can discourage GLBTI people from being open about their sexual orientation or gender identity, which can have significant mental health problems including social isolation and disconnectedness, anxiety and distress (McNair & Medland, 2002). As well as their shared experience of heterosexism, GLBTI people also have their own distinctive social and cultural practices, which may increase their risk factors for a range of health problems—for example, drug and alcohol use, body image (associated with factors such as eating disorders and gym culture) and non-compliance with medication (McNair & Medland, 2002).

As noted earlier, older people are at risk of marginalisation and social exclusion. These processes are exacerbated for GLBTI people who are aged. Consider, for example, the deeply held prejudices that older people should not be sexually active and the impact of these prejudices on people whose sexuality and gender identity is non-normative. Ageing is recognised as a key transitional life period during which access to social support and health and welfare services can help to maintain health and well-being; however, there has been very little research on the health-related needs of GBLTI people as they age (McNair & Harrison, 2002). Research by Chamberlin and Robinson (2002) found that older gay men who were from working-class backgrounds were particularly at risk of marginalisation and social isolation because they are excluded from mainstream society as well as the gay subculture of youth and beauty.

Much of the Australian government aged care policy is embedded within heteronormativity and as such does not acknowledge the diversity that exists around the sexuality and gender identity of older people and how this shapes family and household composition, caring relationships and financial arrangements (Harrison, 2005). Thus, older GLBTI people are concerned about their invisibility within the aged care sector and the loneliness and social isolation that ensues. As a result of this heteronormativity, the prospect of being cared for in an aged-care institution is a major concern for older GLBTI people. The impact of heterosexism is evident in the issues identified by Harrison (1999), which include a fear of emotional and physical abuse; a reduced standard of care because of prejudicial attitudes; a lack of physical intimacy because of taboos against displays of same-sex affection; and intersex people's fear of inappropriate treatment because of anatomical variations. Participants in research by Chamberlin and Robinson (2002) identified the need for nursing homes and retirement villages for non-heterosexual people, although they also acknowledged the logistical difficulties inherent in this proposal.

Question for reflection

How can knowledge of social marginalisation assist health workers to understand the health issues facing GLBTI people?

CONCLUSION

Health issues facing groups in our society who are marginalised or excluded are therefore complex, particularly when we consider the range of case studies presented in this chapter. Studies of health workers reveal that attitudes towards the aged, socially isolated and impoverished may threaten the quality of care that is received, with a common theme in all groups that are socially excluded or marginalised being the need for 'respect' from health workers. With regard to homeless young people (and this may be applied to all groups who face social exclusion or marginalisation), Ensign and Panke

(2002: 166) state: 'Health care providers need to recognise and appreciate the lifestyle, beliefs and adaptive attitudes of homeless youth, rather than labelling them as "deviant"'. This may be the first step in recognising and addressing the social processes that mean some groups are socially excluded or marginalised.

The health consequences of exclusion from society are varied—from loss of self-esteem, to reduced fitness and higher rates of smoking and drinking. While many of these risks may be viewed as individual in nature, giving rise to victim blaming, sociologists have suggested that the idea of agency is not so clear-cut. In their study of nursing students, Reutter et al. (2004: 305) point to the difficulty in moving beyond an attitude of individual responsibility: 'Students, like the public, may be socialised to believe that individual responsibility with an emphasis on health-enhancing behaviours is the cornerstone of health'. Lack of power and control over one's life is, in fact, a structural issue related to being excluded from, or marginalised within, a mainstream world.

REVIEW QUESTIONS

1   What does Saunders (2003: 5) mean when he says: 'In the wrong hands, social exclusion can become a vehicle for vilifying those who do not conform and an excuse for seeing their problems as caused by their own "aberrant behaviour"'?
2   How does social exclusion/social marginalisation affect health for people in each of the four case studies in this chapter? How can health workers practice in a way that minimises the effects of social exclusion or social marginalisation?

KEY TERMS

Active exclusion/passive exclusion
Ageism
Citizenship
Domestic violence
Equality and equity
Gender
Gerontology
Heteronormativity
Heterosexism

Homophobia
Ideology
Poverty
Social death
Social exclusion
Social marginalisation
Stereotype
Transphobia

FURTHER READING

Burdekin, B. 1989, *Our Homeless Children*, Canberra, Human Rights and Equal Opportunities Commission.

Burstein, M. 2005, 'Combating the social exclusion of at-risk groups', Policy Research Initiative Paper, Government of Canada.

Dixon, J. and Welch, N. 2000, 'Researching the rural–metropolitan health differential using the "social determinants of health"', *Australian Journal of Rural Health*, 8, pp. 254–60.

Ensign, J. and Panke, E. 2002, 'Barriers and bridges to care: voices of homeless female adolescent youth in Seattle, Washington, USA', *Journal of Advanced Nursing*, 37, pp. 166–72.

Gray, D.E. 2006, *Health Sociology: An Australian Perspective*, Frenchs Forest, Pearson Education.

Hillier, L. and Harrison, L. 1999, 'The girls in our town: sex, love, relationships and rural life', in La Nauze, H., Briskman, L. and Lynn, M. (eds), *Challenging Rural Practice: Human Services in Australia*, Melbourne, Australian Centre in Sex, Health and Society.

Keleher, H. 2004a, 'Promoting healthy ageing', in Keleher, H. and Murphy, B. (eds), *Understanding Health: A Determinants Approach*, South Melbourne, Oxford University Press, pp. 312–17.

Keleher, H. 2004b, 'Social exclusion', in Keleher, H. and Murphy, B. (eds), *Understanding Health: A Determinants Approach*, South Melbourne, Oxford University Press, pp. 246–51.

Leonard, W. 2002, *What's the Difference? Health Issues of Major Concern to Gay, Lesbian, Bisexual, Transgender and Intersex (GLBTI) Victorians*, Leonard, W. (ed.), Ministerial Advisory Committee on Gay and Lesbian Health, Victorian Government Department of Human Services, Melbourne.

Mission Australia 2005, 'The voices of homeless young Australians, Snapshot 2005', www.missionaustralia.com.au, accessed 15 September 2006.

Saunders, P. 2003, *Can Social Exclusion provide a New Framework for Measuring Poverty?* In Discussion Paper No. 127, Sydney, Social Policy Research Centre.

Sen, A. 2000, *Social Exclusion: Concept, Application and Scrutiny*, Social Development, Paper No. 1, Office of Environment and Social Development, Manila, Asia Development Bank.

Strazzari, M. 2006, 'Ageing, dying and death in the twenty-first century', in Germov, J. (ed.), *Second Opinion: An Introduction to Health Sociology*, South Melbourne, Oxford University Press, pp. 244–64.

Wainer, J. and Chesters, J. 2000, 'Rural mental health: Neither romanticism nor despair', *Australian Journal of Rural Health*, 8, pp. 141–7.

Chapter 7

The Health of Aboriginal and Torres Strait Islander Peoples

Introduction

Last night, a popular current affairs program reported on petrol sniffing among particular communities of Australian Aboriginals. The reporter highlighted the incessant use of inhalants as a way in which some Aboriginal people get 'high' and how this state of being impedes their ability and motivation to get jobs, look after their families and lead civilised lives. Julia and some of her fellow nursing students are discussing their thoughts about the program, which is leading to quite a hot debate. Phoebe, one of Julia's closest friends at university, is upset about the ways the report sensationalised the use of petrol as an intoxicant among Australian Aboriginals and is arguing that television programs should stop continuing to impose negative cultural stereotypes. Phoebe is outnumbered by Ed, Kylie, Samuel and Billy who argue that all individuals have a choice and some Aboriginal people are choosing to sniff petrol and be unemployed. Julia is aware of how contentious the issue of social marginalisation is among Australia's Indigenous population, but she wonders how, as students, she and her classmates should view the dilemma. Are there any considerations missing from these arguments?

Nowhere are the health effects of marginalisation and social exclusion more keenly experienced than in Australia's Aboriginal and Torres Strait Islander peoples. While recent research suggests that their health status may be improving, there remains a vast gap between Aboriginal and Torres Strait Islander peoples and that of other Australians. The health status of Aboriginal people is worse than other Australians on every indicator: life expectancy, maternal mortality, infant mortality, childhood mortality and adult mortality.

Aboriginal and Torres Strait Islander peoples' health disadvantage needs to be considered in the broader context of social disadvantage, inequality and exclusion, political marginalisation and the historical currents of colonialism. A critical sociological approach points to the need to take account of historical, social and cultural factors in order to understand the health disadvantage faced by Aboriginal peoples in contemporary society. This enhances our knowledge of the unequal health outcomes between Aboriginal and non-Aboriginal people by focusing on the impacts of social structure as well as the cultural appropriateness of health care services.

Objectives

After reading this chapter, you should be able to:

■ understand why the history of dispossession and colonisation is the focus of contemporary understanding of Aboriginal health
■ explain how social processes such as marginalisation contribute to poorer health outcomes for Aboriginal peoples
■ critically evaluate the differing approaches to Aboriginal health improvement.

In this chapter we use the term Aboriginal and Torres Strait Islander peoples when referring to the total population of Indigenous Australians (see cultural protocol at the end of the chapter).

Aboriginal and Torres Strait Islander peoples' systems, society and culture

Many myths and misconceptions exist in the general population about the health and lifestyle of Aboriginal and Torres Strait Islander peoples. For example, there is a view that Aboriginal people do not want to work; however, in reality, increasing employment is a widely shared aspiration among Aboriginal people and one consistently advocated by Aboriginal leaders (Bula Ngumbaay Aboriginal Consultants, 2002). This chapter will debunk myths like these by presenting relevant data that more accurately depicts contemporary Aboriginal and Torres Strait Islander society and clearly illustrates patterns of ill health and disadvantage.

In the past, studies of Aboriginal and Torres Strait Islander systems, society and culture have tended towards an ethnocentric viewpoint, whereby the researcher's observations have been interpreted with reference to, and premised on, the superiority of their own systems, society and culture. As a result, Aboriginal and Torres Strait Islander systems, society and culture have been framed as different or 'other', leading to what Anderson (2004: 84) refers to as an 'overemphasis on difference'. Such interpretations were usually negative—for example, whereas the European settlers saw themselves as civilised and hard-working, the Aboriginal people were seen as primitive and lazy. Some of this thinking persists and underpins stereotypes of Aboriginal people.

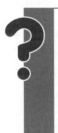

Question for reflection

Think about some of the ways that Aboriginal and Torres Strait Islander peoples are portrayed in the popular media—for example, in current affairs programs, tourism and sport. What are the images that are commonly conveyed?

The persistence of myths, misconceptions and ethnocentric viewpoints are in part confounded by the relatively small number of Aboriginal and Torres Strait Islander peoples living throughout Australia, which is approximately 458,520 (representing just 2.4 per cent of the total Australian population). The diversity that exists within the Aboriginal and Torres Strait Islander population is often overlooked. For example, of the total Indigenous population, approximately 89 per cent are Aboriginal people, 6 per cent are Torres Strait Islanders and 4 per cent are both Aboriginal and Torres Strait Islander peoples (Australian Bureau of Statistics, 2003). Aboriginal people have tended to live on mainland Australia,

Tasmania and the adjacent islands, whereas Torres Strait Islanders came from the islands of the Torres Strait between the tip of Cape York in Queensland and Papua New Guinea. While Aboriginal people have largely remained in the same areas, about 80 per cent of the Torres Strait Islander population now lives outside the Torres Strait. Aboriginal people and Torres Strait Islanders are culturally and ethnically distinct peoples, and their histories since European settlement are also different. However, some of their experiences are similar in respect of the way that they have been subjected to the same restrictive and paternalistic government policies (Aboriginal and Torres Strait Islander Commission, 1999).

The distribution of the Aboriginal and Torres Strait Islander population varies in each state and territory, and is possibly at odds with what is generally believed. The proportion of the Aboriginal and Torres Strait Islander population by state/territory and the distribution by remoteness of area are depicted in Table 7.1 and Figure 7.1 respectively. The highest proportion of the total Aboriginal and Torres Strait Islander population lives in New South Wales (29.4 per cent), closely followed by Queensland (27.4 per cent). A greater proportion of Aboriginal and Torres Strait Islander people live outside major urban centres, compared with other Australians; however, this is not to say that all Indigenous people live in rural or remote areas—in 2001, 30.2 per cent lived in major cities, 27 per cent lived in remote areas, whereas 43 per cent lived in regional areas (Trewin & Madden, 2005).

TABLE 7.1   Estimated resident Indigenous population (30 June 2001)

	Indigenous population	Proportion of total Indigenous population	Proportion of total state/territory population
New South Wales	134,900	29.4%	2.1%
Queensland	125,900	27.5%	3.5%
Northern Territory	56,900	12.4%	28.8%
Victoria	27,800	6.1%	0.6%
South Australia	25,500	5.6%	1.7%
Tasmania	17,400	3.8%	3.7%
Australian Capital Territory	3,900	0.9%	1.2%
Australia (a)	458,500	100%	2.4%

(a)   Includes other Territories

Source: *Experimental Estimates and Projections of Indigenous Australians, 1991 to 2009* (cat. no. 3238.0)
Australian Bureau of Statistics; used with permission from the ABS

FIGURE 7.1   Australian population distribution by Indigenous status (30 June 2001)

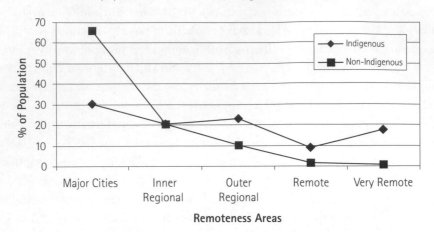

Source: *Year Book of Australia 2004* (cat. no. 1301.0) and *Experimental Estimates and Projections of Indigenous Australians, 1991 to 2009* (cat. no. 3238.0) Australian Bureau of Statistics 2004b; used with permission from the ABS

Historical context: from traditional through transitional to contemporary

Grant Sarra Consultancy Services (n.d.) suggests that Aboriginal systems, society and culture have evolved over three important stages: traditional (pre-1788); transitional (post-1788); and contemporary (1967–now).

The traditional stage

Traditional Aboriginal systems are complex and relate to all facets of life, including coexistence with others; kinship; roles of men, women and children; lore; and punishment. Their spirituality includes beliefs about ancestral beings, the time of creation, and ceremonies and rituals for life events such as birth, deaths and marriages. There is a strong oral tradition to convey, perpetuate and promulgate history, education and customs, which were often told as stories. There were many (some estimate as many as 500) different Aboriginal groups with their own languages, kinship ties and culture. There are complex social systems about the relationship of these groups with the land, involving both rights and duties—rights to use the land and its products, and duties to tend the land through the performance of ceremonies. Failure to observe the laws of the land and interference with its spiritual places has consequences not only for the land, but also for the people charged with its maintenance (Aboriginal and Torres Strait Islander Commission, 1999). A part of this strong connection to the land, animals and environment is the notion that the people belong to the land and life is a shared existence. This extended to a system of sharing and reciprocity.

The transitional era

During the transitional era, the traditional Aboriginal systems, society and culture were disrupted. What is recorded as 'settlement' in European history books can also be viewed as an 'invasion'. The European invaders (settlers) came to Australia informed by their scientific beliefs and theories about colonisation and indigenous inhabitants. These included theories about the origin and nature of humankind such as the great chain of being theory and social Darwinism, which assumed that white-skinned Europeans were physically, intellectually and culturally superior. These pseudo-scientific beliefs were coupled with xenophobia (a morbid fear of foreigners) and a strong Protestant work ethic. 'On the basis of these perceived superior values and pseudoscientific beliefs, it was thought by the dominant group that Aborigines had no culture, no morality, no religion, no soul, no humanity, and that by a process of natural selection, they would die out' (Eckerman et al., 1992 in Smith, 2004: 23). Thus, there was no recognition of the Aboriginal peoples' prior existence, social structure, kinship system, values and beliefs or the traditional value of land, plants and the environment. It was this set of values, beliefs and theories that allowed the dispossession of Aboriginal land, the institutionalisation of racism and the enforcement of paternalistic and restrictive policies.

In addition to the threat to health and well-being as a result of introduced diseases, the Aboriginal peoples' access to traditional foods and traditional way of life was also threatened. The failure to account for Aboriginal systems, society and culture is most evident in the way the European invaders dealt with their relationships with land and their family. Unlike other countries that were explored during the period of colonisation, Australia was declared as terra nullius—land belonging to no one, the ownership of which in international law can therefore be claimed by another nation (Australians for Native Title and Reconciliation, 2004). Some Aboriginal people were forcibly removed from the land with which they had particular spiritual connections, others had to accommodate those who had been forced off their traditional land. As well as removal from their land, Aboriginal children were forcibly separated from their families in accordance with various 'protectionist' policies. A range of high-profile reports and investigations have served to raise awareness and begin to address the consequences of these actions.

The following is an excerpt from National Report of the Royal Commission into Aboriginal Deaths in Custody (Johnston, E. QC, 1991, Volume 1, Section 1.4—The Importance of History, copyright of Commonwealth of Australia, reproduced by permission):

That Aboriginal people were dispossessed of their land without benefit of treaty, agreement or compensation is generally known. But I think little known is the amount of brutality and bloodshed that was involved in enforcing on the ground what was pronounced by the law. Aboriginal people were deprived of their land and if they showed resistance they were summarily dealt with. The loss of land meant the destruction of the Aboriginal economy which everywhere was based upon hunting and foraging. And the land use adopted by the settlers drastically reduced the population of animals to be hunted and plants to be foraged. And the loss of the land threatened the Aboriginal culture which all over Australia was based upon land and relationship to the land. These were the most dramatic effects of European colonisation supplemented by the decimating effects of introduced disease to which the Aboriginal people had no resistance ...

Having reduced the original inhabitants to a condition, in many places, of abject dependency the colonial governments decided upon a policy of protection which had two main thrusts: Aboriginal people were swept up into reserves and missions where they were supervised as to every detail of their lives and there was a deliberate policy of undermining and destroying their spiritual and cultural beliefs. The other aspect of that policy as it developed was that Aboriginal children of mixed race descent—usually Aboriginal mother and non-Aboriginal father—were removed from their family and the land, placed in institutions and trained to grow up as good European labourers or domestics ...

The theory was that the 'full blood' Aboriginal people would die out and they should be provided with a little care while they did so; and that the 'mixed blood' would be bred out. When these expectations proved ill founded, another policy was tried, that of assimilation. But the old supervisor remained in place; in the Northern Territory Aboriginal people remained wards of the State, in the States the Protectorate and the Boards remained in place with all their powers, children continued to be removed but the whole aim was now to assimilate the Aboriginal people by encouraging them to accept the Western culture and lifestyle, give up their culture, become culturally absorbed and indistinguishable, other than physically, from the dominant group. For a short time, integration replaced assimilation as the policy option with little change in any practical way. And that was the practice in 1967 when the Referendum was carried which gave power to the Commonwealth to make laws relating to Aboriginal people ...

... Every turn in the policy of government and the practice of the non-Aboriginal community was postulated on the inferiority of the Aboriginal people; the original expropriation of their land was based on the idea that the land was not occupied and the people uncivilised; the protection policy was based on the view that Aboriginal people could not achieve a place in the non-Aboriginal society and that they must be protected against themselves while the race died out; the assimilationist policy assumed that their culture and way of life is without value and that we confer a favour on them by assimilating them into our ways; even to the point of taking their children and removing them from family.

... I do not suggest, of course, that many non-Aboriginal people have not been guided by the best of motives; and in point of fact some missions and probably some reserves offered an opportunity for some Aboriginal people to maintain their unity and a measure of cohesion at a time when this might have been threatened in the larger society. But all this was done in the sure knowledge that the people needed our superior skills and ideas.

Contemporary: linking the past to the present

The characteristics of contemporary Aboriginal systems, society and culture can only be understood in respect of their history. Studies of Aboriginal and Torres Strait Islander peoples' culture and language have found that those living in remote areas are more likely to have stronger cultural attachments. For example, an Indigenous language is the main language spoken at home for 39 per cent of Aboriginal and Torres Strait Islander peoples living in remote areas, compared with only 2 per cent of those living in non-remote areas (Trewin & Madden, 2005). As a result, there is a view that the Aboriginal and Torres Strait Islander peoples who live in remote areas are more 'authentic' than their urban counterparts. However, this viewpoint ignores the temporal nature of culture. Just as other cultures have changed over time, so have Aboriginal and Torres Strait Islander cultures. There is a diversity of Aboriginal and Torres Strait Islander cultures throughout Australia (Aboriginal and Torres Strait Islander Commission, 1999).

The cultural diversity that exists among Aboriginal and Torres Strait Islander peoples is reflected in the variety of understandings of health and illness. While there is little information about the contemporary health beliefs of the Aboriginal population, especially those living in urban areas (Maher, 1999), it is generally acknowledged that the traditional health beliefs of Aboriginal peoples remain an important influence on health beliefs and ideas today.

Western perspectives of health and illness are vastly different from traditional beliefs of Aboriginal and Torres Strait Islander peoples. Even the word 'health', as Westerners know it, does not exist in many Aboriginal languages (National Aboriginal Health Strategy Working Party, 1989).

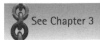 See Chapter 3

Informed by knowledge passed from the traditional stage, health is viewed as just one part of life that is interconnected with many other parts of life, such as the land, kinship obligations and religion. Health and well-being are achieved through meeting these social and spiritual obligations. The National Aboriginal Health Strategy Working Party explains that 'Health is not just the physical well-being of the individual but the social, emotional and cultural well-being of the whole community. This is a whole-of-life view and it includes the cyclical concept of life–death–life' (1989). Traditional understandings about why people get sick revolve around the role of the environment, social relationships and, in particular, the supernatural that 'provides the explanations of "why me" and

"why now", which is unable to be answered in terms of Western medical theory'
(Maher, 1999: 231).

Question for reflection

In what ways do traditional understandings of the causes of Aboriginal
and Torres Strait Islander peoples' poor health differ from Western views
of health and illness?

The health impacts of history, society and culture

It is difficult to piece together an accurate picture of Aboriginal and Torres Strait
Islander peoples' health in Australia because of the lack of comprehensive data.
Although Aboriginal and Torres Strait Islander peoples' health disadvantages
have been recognised for many years prior, a national policy requiring the
collection of statistics about the health of the Indigenous population was not
formulated until 1973 (Thomson, 2003). The Australian Institute of Health and
Welfare (AIHW) reports that the data about Aboriginal and Torres Strait Islander
people are limited by the extent to which Indigenous people are included in
national surveys, the accuracy with which they are identified in both surveys and
administrative datasets, uncertainties about Indigenous population estimates,
and concerns about whether the survey methods employed are always the most
suitable (Trewin & Madden, 2005). The Northern Territory is reported to have
the best data collection and, by comparison, there is relatively little information
known about Aboriginals in other states and territories. With these limitations in
mind, information about Aboriginal and Torres Strait Islander health and social
well-being is presented in Table 7.2.

TABLE 7.2   Selected indicators of Aboriginal and Torres Strait Islander health and social well-being

Life expectancy	The probability of a 20 year old person dying before his or her 55th birthday is two to six times higher for Indigenous Australians.
	In the period 1996–2001, the life expectancy at birth was estimated at 59 years for Indigenous males and 65 years for Indigenous females, well below the 77 years for all Australian males and 82 years for all Australian females in 1998–2000.

Infant mortality	The proportion of births to Indigenous mothers that are low birth weight is twice the rate observed in non-Indigenous mothers.
	The infant mortality rate in selected jurisdictions, despite showing declines over the last 10 years, continues to be three times that of the non-Indigenous population.
Adult mortality	Death rates from diabetes are between seven and 20 times as high as the rates in the non-Indigenous population.
	Death rates from circulatory disease in the Indigenous population are four to five times the rate in the non-Indigenous population.
	Death rates from respiratory diseases are between five and six times as high, and death rates from lung cancer are between two and three times as high.
	Indigenous people die from injury at between two and four times the rates of non-Indigenous people.
	Mortality from self-harm is two to four times the rate in the non-Indigenous population, and morbidity is two to three times as high.
Adult morbidity	Hospitalisation rates for depressive and anxiety disorders are between one and three times the rates in the non-Indigenous population.
	Rates of infection with Chlamydia, *gonococcus* and syphilis are also high.
	Indigenous people are hospitalised for injury at between three and four times the rates of non-Indigenous people.
Health risk factors	Approximately 48 per cent of Indigenous adults are overweight or obese.
	Approximately 53 per cent of Indigenous adults are current smokers.
	Approximately 69 per cent of Indigenous adults consume alcohol and of those who do, 50 per cent consumed it at risky or high-risk levels in the last 12 months.
	The rate of hospitalisation for substance use disorders is five to eight times higher in the Indigenous population.
Income	Seventy-six per cent of Indigenous households had an adjusted weekly income below the 50th percentile, compared to 52 per cent of non-Indigenous households.
Education	In 2002, the proportion of Indigenous males and females aged 20–24 years who had completed year 12 or equivalent was less than half of that for non-Indigenous males and females (27 per cent compared with 64 per cent and 29 per cent compared with 73 per cent respectively).
Employment	In 2002, 52 per cent of Indigenous people aged 20–64 years were employed in full-time or part-time work, 12 per cent were unemployed and 36 per cent were not in the labour force. The comparison figures for the non-Indigenous population were 75 per cent, 4 per cent and 21 per cent respectively.

Source: Standing Committee on Aboriginal and Torres Strait Islander Health and Statistical Information Management Committee, 2006; data used with permission from the Australian Institute of Health and Welfare

Question for reflection

What does the information in Table 7.2 tell us about the links between health and social well-being for Aboriginal peoples?

Aboriginal peoples are disadvantaged compared to other Australians on a range of health and social indicators. In 2002, the real mean equalised gross household income of Indigenous people was equal to 59 per cent of that of non-Indigenous adults (Trewin & Madden, 2005). The lack of educational and life opportunities is interlinked with a complex array of health and social outcomes. For example, Aboriginal and Torres Strait Islander peoples are over-represented in the justice system (Indigenous people were imprisoned at eleven times the rate of other Australians), and experience higher rates of alcohol and substance abuse and family violence (Standing Committee on Aboriginal and Torres Strait Islander Health and Statistical Information Management Committee, 2006). Trewin and Madden (2005) also identify links between self-assessed health status and removal from families, with 39 per cent of males and 41 per cent of females removed from families reporting fair or poor health compared with 21 per cent of males and 22 per cent of females who had not been removed. Consider also the links between cultural attachment and self-assessed health status, with higher levels of fair or poor health reported for those Aboriginals who spoke English as their main language at home than for those who spoke an Aboriginal or Torres Strait Islander language at home (Trewin & Madden, 2005).

See Chapter 6

The social and economic disadvantage of Aboriginal and Torres Strait Islander peoples can be understood using the concept of marginalisation. Here, marginalisation is understood as 'separation and alienation from work relations, family and other social relations that bind people into communities and give value to lives' (Aboriginal and Torres Strait Islander Commission, 1999: 64), pointing to marginalisation as a product of Aboriginal and Torres Strait Islander peoples' history outlined above where they were positioned as outsiders and inferior, and were subject to policies and practices that exacerbated their outsider status. It is also claimed that 'marginalisation gives rise to self-destructive behaviour, including alcohol and other substance abuse, intra-community violence and crime' (Aboriginal and Torres Strait Islander Commission, 1999: 64).

Addressing health issues: different approaches, different solutions

Part of the key to addressing the health problems facing Aboriginal and Torres Strait Islander peoples is to recognise that they are not inevitable and that they are preventable. Critics argue that the issues relating to the health and well-being of the Aboriginal and Torres Strait Islander peoples have been well researched and documented, and that the time for action is overdue. The following section highlights how solutions for the problems facing Aboriginal and Torres Strait Islander peoples are framed differently according to the way that these problems are explained.

Health care provision through an individualistic approach

When health problems are explained in terms of individual biology, the result is solutions such as the provision of one-to-one care and treatment. Explaining poor health in terms of lifestyle or risk factors leads to a focus on individual attributes. These approaches also tend to lapse into victim blaming, which in turn serves to perpetuate stereotypes and racial discrimination. For example, for many years it was believed that Aboriginal people were biologically less able to handle alcohol until the 'fire water theory' was refuted in 1991 (Hunter et al., 1991). Yet the commonly held views that there is a genetic contributing factor, all Aboriginal people are drinkers and all Aboriginal people who drink are drunks persist despite the evidence to the contrary. The National Aboriginal Health Strategy Working Party (1989: 194) stated: 'there is consensus in the Aboriginal community that understands the "alcohol problem" from a community perspective, as a symptom (ultimately a symptom of dispossession) of alienation, and discrimination which leads to loss of self esteem'. Thus, with a focus on individual biology, the broader social, economic and environmental factors are generally ignored. There is a lack of recognition that the provision of health services alone will not improve Aboriginal and Torres Strait Islander health.

   When health solutions are located in the provision of health care services, Western (biomedical) ideas about health and illness tend to prevail. As a result, Aboriginal and Torres Strait Islander peoples' experience of the health system involves negotiating two cultures—their own and the dominant culture of a system based on a very different view of health. Thus, the dominance of Western cultural values poses a major barrier to Aboriginal and Torres Strait Islander peoples in accessing mainstream health systems.

Different types of health care services: the primary health care approach

As can be seen from the following statement about health, Aboriginal and Torres Strait Islander peoples take a much broader view of their health problems and the solutions that are required.

Health to Aboriginal peoples is a matter of determining all aspects of their life, including control over their physical environment, of dignity, of community self-esteem, and of justice. It is not merely a matter of the provision of doctors, hospitals, medicines or the absence of disease and incapacity. (National Aboriginal Health Strategy Working Party, 1989)

Successful approaches to the provision of health care to Aboriginal and Torres Strait Islander peoples have been based on primary health care principles. A primary health care approach includes a focus on health promotion and prevention, as well as community participation. The National Aboriginal and Torres Strait Islander Health Strategy has a strong emphasis on supporting the development of comprehensive community-controlled primary health care services. International experience shows that the involvement of Indigenous people in the delivery of education and health care programs contributes to improvements in the health of themselves, their families and communities. The Aboriginal and Torres Strait Islander Health Workforce National Strategic Framework (Standing Committee on Aboriginal and Torres Strait Islander Health, 2002) has been developed with the aim of transforming and consolidating the workforce in Aboriginal and Torres Strait Islander health and is underpinned by the following principles: cultural respect; a holistic approach; health sector responsibility; community control of primary health care services; working together; localised decision making; promoting good health; building the capacity of health services and communities; and accountability for health outcomes.

Examples of the Aboriginal and Torres Strait Islander health workforce include Aboriginal Health Workers and Indigenous registered nurses. Aboriginal Health Workers complete either a Certificate III or IV in Aboriginal Primary Health Care Practice, which equips them with the knowledge and skills to function as a primary health care practitioner and deliver holistic health care, which may include clinical care, health promotion or community development. However, currently, only the Northern Territory has a registration system in place for Aboriginal Health Workers as their role and scope is contested in other states and territories of Australia. There are national projects, such as the Indigenous Nursing Education Working Group (2002), that have been developed to increase the number of registered Aboriginal and Torres Strait Islander nurses, as well as promoting the integration of Indigenous health issues into core nursing curricula.

Allocation of resources

Explanations of Aboriginal and Torres Strait Islander health and well-being that highlight contextual issues, such as political and economic factors, emphasise the role of inequality. Such analyses explore the role of poverty, allocation of health funding and distribution of health services in determining health status. For example, Gray and Saggers (2005) focus on the roles of public health infrastructure and health system funding. It is well documented that inadequate housing, water, sewerage and electricity are associated with higher rates of poor health and infectious diseases. Only in New South Wales, Victoria and Tasmania are all permanent dwellings (1397 of the total 16,649 dwellings throughout Australia) in discrete Indigenous communities connected to sewerage, water and electricity. Although the majority of permanent dwellings had these amenities, there were still 301 without an organised sewerage system, 147 without an organised water supply and 257 without electricity (Standing Committee on Aboriginal and Torres Strait Islander Health and Statistical Information Management Committee, 2006).

Many reports about the health and well-being of Aboriginal and Torres Strait Islander peoples refer to the problematic nature of the allocation of responsibilities and funding for Indigenous health between federal and state governments. International comparisons from countries such as New Zealand and Canada, where Indigenous health has significantly improved, point to the pivotal role of federal government responsibility in providing coordinated health services and improved access to resources and infrastructure. In Australia, responsibility for health funding is shared between federal and state/territory governments, thus no one level of government has total responsibility for the health problems. There is a call for greater coordination between federal and state and territory governments, as well as an increase in expenditure. In 2001–02, spending on Indigenous health represented 2.8 per cent of the total national health expenditure. 'The average expenditure per person was $3901 per Indigenous person compared to $3308 per person spent on all other Australians—a ratio of $1.18 for every $1 spent on other Australians' (Standing Committee on Aboriginal and Torres Strait Islander Health and Statistical Information Management Committee, 2006: xvii). There is thus an apparent contradiction between the amount of money spent per person, and the continuing poor health status and outcomes of Aboriginal and Torres Strait Islander peoples. This suggests that in addition to more expenditure, we need to critically examine the appropriateness of those services that are provided, as well as to locate solutions in the broader social determinants of health.

Beyond health care services: towards social and political solutions

Those who emphasise the importance of history and colonisation appreciate the holistic nature of the health and well-being of Aboriginal and Torres Strait Islander peoples and advocate strongly for land rights, self-determination and reconciliation. As mentioned earlier in this chapter, land ownership is viewed by

Aboriginal and Torres Strait Islander peoples as fundamental to their health and well-being. Inquiries into Aboriginal land issues have been high profile and highly contentious. The most significant of these is the Mabo case, which took place in the High Court of Australia in 1992. The High Court rejected the doctrine of terra nullius and recognised Indigenous rights and interests in the land. Shortly after this verdict, the *Native Title Act 1993* was enacted to provide a legislative framework for native title. Legislation granting Aboriginal groups' interests in land varies from state to state and currently about 20 per cent has been returned to traditional ownership. The objective of land acquisition is to provide a base for economic, social and cultural development. It is important to note that land returned to traditional ownership is communally owned, not privately owned by individuals, consistent with a view of the land as having spiritual rather than commercial value.

Since the 1967 Referendum, when Australians voted to enable the Australian Government to legislate in relation to Aboriginal peoples and for their inclusion in national censuses, Aboriginal and Torres Strait Islander peoples have had some influence in policy development. In the 1970s, the Australian Government adopted self-determination as a policy. The intent of self-determination in relation to the International Covenant on Civil and Political Rights (ICCPR) is to recognise the inherent right of distinct peoples to make decisions about the full range of fundamental freedoms and human rights of indigenous peoples. It has resulted in the creation of self-managing Aboriginal and Torres Strait Islander institutions and organisations, such as Aboriginal Legal Aid and Aboriginal Medical Services. Aboriginal-controlled health services have significantly improved health care and health outcomes for Aboriginal and Torres Strait Islander peoples. The National Aboriginal and Torres Strait Islander Health Strategy and the Healing Hands: Indigenous Health Rights provide examples of these. However, there is no current recognition that Aboriginal and Torres Strait Islander peoples are fully autonomous peoples. This has resulted in some debate about the extent to which the practice of self-determination is accorded to Aboriginal and Torres Strait Islander peoples because it has not been accompanied by decision-making power, as is shown in the following:

> Accordingly, self determination, considered as a component of the Commonwealth social justice policy, is not a matter of right: when finally reduced, it is a welfare measure directed at Aboriginal and Torres Strait Islander peoples. It may accord a far greater degree of respect and dignity to our peoples than past welfare measures. But it nonetheless rests on a policy decision taken by the Commonwealth Government *about us*. It does not recognise our collective right, as distinct peoples. (Dodson, 1993, original emphasis)

Another contentious issue relating to the health and well-being of Aboriginal and Torres Strait Islander peoples is the issue of reconciliation. Reconciliation is a process of reparation and comprises an acknowledgment and apology; guarantees against repetition, measures of restitution, measures of rehabilitation; and monetary compensation (Jackson & Ward, 1999). The issue arose in 1997 from a National Inquiry into the Separation of Aboriginal and Torres Strait Islander Children from their Families (Human Rights and Equal Opportunity Commission) that called for an apology from all Australian parliaments, churches, police forces and other non-government agencies that were involved in the administration of the laws and policies (Smith, 2004). From the perspective that Aboriginal peoples are a marginalised group in our society, reconciliation is seen as critical to addressing some of the effects of social marginalisation, particularly in the areas of health, housing and education. Advocates for reconciliation claim that it enables the nation to move forward with improving outcomes for Aboriginal peoples in a way that is respectful and recognises the effects of past policies and practices.

Towards health rights for Aboriginal and Torres Strait Isiander peoples

As can be seen, the issues are complex and no one solution in itself will suffice. However, it is well known that the imposition of a model of health, even if adequately funded, that does not take account of the particular health needs of Aboriginal and Torres Strait Islander peoples along with understanding their ideas, values and culture—as well as the effects of their marginalised status in Australian society—will not redress the social and health disadvantages that are endemic in this group in our population. The following Health Rights Statement may provide a useful basis for exploring how best to address health issues for Aboriginal and Torres Strait Islander peoples:

Indigenous Health Rights Statement

The health of Indigenous Australians is the worst in the developed world. Indigenous infants die at nearly three times the rate of other Australian infants; their lives will, on average be twenty years shorter; and they are much more likely to suffer chronic disease.

In a wealthy country like Australia gross inequality and neglect is shameful and abhorrent. It is also preventable. In similar countries, such as Canada, New Zealand and the United States, the health of Indigenous people has been rapidly improved by determined and concerted government action.

The necessary first step in resolving the present crisis in Australia is to recognise that it is not inevitable.

Australia must acknowledge that the crisis began with colonisation and dispossession and became endemic when social and economic disadvantage became entrenched. The crisis will not end until these conditions are changed.

If the health of Indigenous Australians is to be improved all Australian governments must resolve to provide:

Primary health care on the basis of need, through Aboriginal community controlled health services and better access to mainstream services;

A significant increase in the health workforce, particularly of Indigenous background;

Comprehensive early intervention and prevention programs;

Significant improvements in educational and employment outcomes, and housing and infrastructure provision.

Health refers not only to the physical well being of individuals, but also to the social, emotional, spiritual and cultural well being of the communities in which they live. It is a commonplace of medical knowledge that poor health is related to social disadvantage; to stress, social exclusion, unemployment and discrimination. Drug use, alcohol dependence and domestic violence are familiar and inevitable parts of the same cycle.

It follows that measures to improve the health of Indigenous Australians must include the application of principles of self-determination on which durable and resourceful communities absolutely depend. Governments must adopt an enabling role in relation to Indigenous governance.

Australia must recognise that the health of Indigenous organisations and communities and the health of Indigenous people are inseparable. It is equally true that improvements in health depend on overturning the destructive legacies of dispossession, including those that relate to land and culture; and the attainment of a secure and valued place for Indigenous peoples in the life of the nation.

(Australians for Native Title and Reconciliation, 2004)

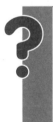

Questions for reflection

What are the elements of a sociological perspective on health and illness that are evident in the Indigenous Health Rights Statement? How useful is a sociological perspective in understanding the issues faced by Aboriginal and Torres Strait Islander peoples?

Following the debate between Phoebe, Ed, Kylie, Samuel and Billy, Julia felt as if she needed to reach some conclusions for herself about the contentious issues raised by the current affairs program, and subsequently discussed by her classmates. She printed the transcript of the current affairs program from the Internet and went to the university library to explore further some of the topics covered in the lecture about the health of Aboriginal and Torres Strait Islander peoples.

Julia can now see the relationships between health disadvantage and other issues, such as social exclusion, inequality, marginalisation and colonialism. Julia understands that these are the same historical, social and cultural factors that shape health and illness experiences that form a critical sociological approach. But she is still interested in the idea that petrol sniffing is a response to social marginalisation, rather than a hedonistic act of stupidity, which is how the current affairs program described it. In the library, Julia finds a great book called *Heavy Metal: The Social Meaning of Petrol Sniffing in Australia*, by Maggie Brady (1992).

Julia discovers in the book that petrol sniffing is often interpreted as a response to 'individual' issues, which aligns with the argument proposed by Ed, Kylie, Samuel and Billy, but that dispossession, rapid social change and colonisation are processes that can offer an additional explanation, such as that held by Phoebe. But Julia also finds out that emphasising one explanation over the other presents a potential problem. While historical, social and cultural factors have shaped the lives of the Indigenous Australian population, an overemphasis on these factors may also lead us to 'victim blame' petrol sniffers for being passive victims of colonisation. If the act of petrol sniffing can't be attributed to individual choices or external factors, how can we explain it?

After a few hours researching, Julia realises that although victim blaming individuals is not the answer, people like Ed, Kylie, Samuel and Billy need to consider that many people of the Indigenous Australian population are socially marginalised. This level of exclusion from society is intrinsically interlinked with the fact that Aboriginal and Torres Strait Islanders have not shared, and to a large extent continue not to share, the same life opportunities as other Australians.

Julia now feels prepared to engage in further conversations on the topic of petrol sniffing. She writes a list of questions that may help her classmates to reflect critically on their opinions.

Questions

1   What are the processes that have led to the overall social marginalisation of Australia's Indigenous population? How do these processes continue to exclude Aboriginal and Torres Strait Islander peoples today?

2   How are negative cultural stereotypes perpetuated in the media? Can you think of other social issues that are often portrayed as characterising Aboriginal and Torres Strait Islander peoples?

3   Why does the emphasis on historical, social and cultural factors as a reason for substance abuse among Australia's Indigenous population, over individual factors, present a problem? How can this be overcome?

Cultural protocol

The term Indigenous is increasingly used to refer to people who are native to a country or have a historical continuity with a society prior to colonisation. For example, the term appears at United Nations Forums, such as the Working Group on Indigenous Populations. In Australia, it is often used to refer collectively to Aboriginal and Torres Strait Islander peoples. As authors of this chapter, our aim is to portray the issues related to the health and well-being of Aboriginal and Torres Strait Islander peoples in a way that is culturally sensitive and politically aware. To this end we acknowledge that Australia has two Indigenous peoples: Aboriginal people and Torres Strait Islanders. We understand that there is significant ethnic and cultural diversity within and between Aboriginal and Torres Strait Islander peoples. For this reason, we have chosen not to use the term Indigenous Australians as it does not denote or respect the difference between the two groups. The term only appears where it is used within other work quoted or referred to in this chapter.

For more information, we encourage you to consult the references for this chapter, which have been compiled with a bias towards authors who are Aboriginal or Torres Strait Islander and with reference to the Aboriginal and Torres Strait Islander protocols for libraries, archives and information services.

CONCLUSION

Aboriginal people still suffer disproportionately from some of the consequences of European settlement, particularly in relation to infectious diseases, chronic illness and social location (Trewin & Madden, 2005). The data presented in this chapter clearly demonstrates the poorer health status of Aboriginal and Torres Strait Islander peoples. The social and economic disadvantage experienced by Aboriginal and Torres Strait Islander peoples contributes to the poor health of many groups of these people. A sociological perspective on the health of Aboriginal people points to the issue of marginalisation within the broader community. The health outcomes of social marginalisation may arise from poverty, unemployment and discrimination, but they are linked also to the history of dispossession and colonisation.

REVIEW QUESTIONS

1   How can a sociological understanding of Aboriginal health result in better informed policies and practices?
2   What does self-determination mean? Why is it contentious? How can it be used as a concept to inform better health for Aboriginal peoples?
3   Why has there been an emphasis on the need for reconciliation in order to improve health and welfare outcomes for Aboriginal peoples?

KEY TERMS

Ethnocentric   Self-determination
Marginalisation   Stereotypes
Reconciliation   Xenophobia

FURTHER READING

Aboriginal and Torres Strait Islander Commission 1999, *As Matter of Fact: Answering the Myths and Misconceptions about Indigenous Australians*, Canberra, Commonwealth of Australia.

Anderson, I. 2004, 'Aboriginal health' in Grbich, C. (ed.), *Health in Australia: Sociological Concepts and Issues*, Frenchs Forest, Pearson Education.

Australians for Native Title and Reconciliation 2004, *Healing Hands: Indigenous Health Rights Action Kit*, Rozelle, ANTaR <www.antar.org.au>.

Dodson, M. 1993, *Aboriginal and Torres Strait Islander Social Justice Commission First Report 1993, Human Rights and Equal Opportunity Commission*, Canberra, Reconciliation and Social Justice Library.

Indigenous Nursing Education Working Group 2002, *'getting em n keepin em'*, Commonwealth Department of Health and Ageing Office for Aboriginal and Torres Strait Islander Health, Canberra.

Johnston, E. 1991, *Royal Commission into Aboriginal Deaths in Custody: National Report Volume 1*, Reconciliation and Social Justice Library, www.austlii.edu.au/au/special/rsjproject/rsjlibrary/rciadic/.

Maher, P. 1999, 'A review of "traditional" Aboriginal health beliefs', *Australian Journal of Rural Health*, 7, pp. 229–36.

Smith, J.D. 2004, *Australia's Rural and Remote Health: A Social Justice Perspective*, Tertiary Press, Croydon.

Thomson, N. 2003, 'The need for Indigenous health information', in Thomson, N. (ed.), *The Health of Indigenous Australians*, South Melbourne, Oxford University Press, pp. 1–24.

Trewin, D. and Madden, R. 2005, *The Health and Welfare of Australia's Aboriginal and Torres Strait Islander Peoples*, ABS cat. no. 4704.0, AIHW cat. no. IHW14, Canberra, Australian Bureau of Statistics and Australian Institute of Health and Welfare.

University Department of Rural Health, Indigenous Health Website, University of Tasmania, www.ruralhealth.utas.edu.au/indigenous-health/.

Part 3

Experiencing Health and Illness

In Part 3 we seek to reveal the links between our experiences of health and illness and social ideas surrounding risk, healthy living and lifestyle. By exploring the way that social processes shape our experiences, we come to understand why people engage in particular health practices. The diversity of health and illness experiences presented in this part highlights the ways in which interactions between health practitioners and their clients are profoundly influenced by dominant social values and beliefs about the 'normal healthy body', biomedicine and the use of technology.

The differential experiences of health and illness are evident in the first chapter of this part, 'The Body, Health and Lifestyle'. This chapter begins with an exploration of the social factors that influence our sense of self then leads into a discussion about how the body in contemporary society has become a site of risk. Through case studies of disability and obesity, we become aware of the ways that the social construction of the 'normal healthy body' determines how we understand ourselves and our place in society. This theme is further explored in Chapter 9, 'The Illness Experience: Chronic Illness' as we examine the influence of chronic illness on individual identity and the consequent social implications. A case study of mental illness illustrates the impact of stigma. The final chapter in this part, 'Contemporary Debates about Health and Illness', discusses the ways that technology shapes our experience of health and illness. We present examples of technologies that are contested to raise the social implications of the proliferation, widespread acceptance and use of health technologies.

Chapter 8

The Body, Health and Lifestyle

Introduction

Experiences of health and illness are shaped by many factors—from ideas about health and health actions, to the social structuring of health experience, as well as the capacity of the health care system to define and treat illness. Public health messages are an important source of health knowledge, informing us about what we should do to stay healthy, as well as about possible signs and symptoms of ill health. However, the line between health and illness is often not clear—current emphasis on risks and risk factors means that our health knowledge and health practices may be based more on social and expert knowledges than on our own feelings of ill health.

In this chapter, we explore some of the issues of 'health' in contemporary society by drawing attention on the sociology of the body. We argue that the body is an important focus of identity construction in contemporary society, which has occurred in a global context where our lives are permeated by ideas about risk and uncertainty. Thus, body work is an important way in which we attempt to gain control and certainty. We conclude by examining the case study of obesity—while it may be self-evident that being overweight is bad for you, a sociological analysis explores the way that our knowledge of obesity is the result of dominant social ideas and highlights the lack of attention to the social patterning of obesity.

Objectives

After reading this chapter, you should be able to:

- critically examine the importance of the 'body' in contemporary ideas about experiences of health and illness
- explore the ways that a public health approach to lifestyle resonates with contemporary ideas about individuals and their bodies
- evaluate the extent to which ideas about the 'normal healthy body' are socially constructed and the impact that this has on health.

The body and social identity

See Chapter 2

As discussed in Chapter 2, the way that the body is understood in medicine is as a biological machine. Sociologists, however, regard the body as a 'socio-cultural construction; that is the ways in which we understand and experience the body are mediated through social, cultural and political processes' (Lupton, 2005: 196). Thus, in order to understand the relationship of the body to ideas about health and illness, we should start by reflecting on our experience of our own bodies.

Exercise: the body and identity

Concentrate on your own body and consider how it is a reflection of who you are. Think about your appearance right now: how does your choice of hairstyle, what you are wearing, the way you are sitting, say about you and your identity? How do you feel about your body? Are you happy with its size, shape, flexibility, mobility? Are there aspects of your body that you particularly like or dislike? What are they and why do you have those feelings about them?

It is interesting to reflect on the degree to which our sense of self and identity is embodied; how our self-conscious perceptions of who we are in the world are inextricably linked with our material bodies. Our gender identities are formed by the degree to which we measure up with the normative ideals of femininity and masculinity, as they are constructed in dominant social ideas about the female and male body.

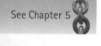
See Chapter 5

In a classic essay titled 'Throwing Like a Girl', Iris Marion Young (1990) describes the ways in which gendered behaviour is embodied. She argues that females develop their bodily practices and behaviours as objects of the 'male gaze'; women conceive of themselves as the object of motion rather than its originator; and women's social existence as the object of the gaze of another is the major source of their bodily self-reference. She explains that 'not only is there a typical style of throwing like a girl, but there is a more or less typical style of running like a girl, climbing like a girl' (Young, 1990: 146). As a result, on commencing a task, women are frequently self-conscious about appearing awkward and at the same time do not want to appear too strong. By contrast, men's embodiment has reinforced the dominant discourse of masculinity being defined in terms of hardness, strength and physical competence, a masculinity that is encapsulated in a readiness to 'risk the body in performance'. These social constructions of femininity and masculinity highlight the centrality of the body in our definitions of who we are.

Our social class, culture and ethnicity may also be represented in the fundamental differences in our everyday bodily practices and experiences. Through the concept of *habitus*, Bourdieu (1984) explores the ways that our bodies contain and reflect a certain cultural capital that is expressed through particular bodily practices. Thus we can say we have bodies, we are bodies and we act with our bodies. Taking a sociological view of the body enables exploration of the way that bodily practices reflect the organisation and power relations of the society in which we live. In this way our bodies provide the site through which social norms and conventions are grounded and regulated. These examples of gender, social class, culture and ethnicity illustrate the concept of 'embodiment'—the 'lived experience of both being a body and having a body' (Lupton, 2005: 196).

Question for reflection

Reflect on your own embodiment—how is your experience of being a body and having a body impacted upon by your gender, class, ethnicity or culture?

Health, medicine and the body

Ideas about the body have become a central feature of the sociological study of health and illness because the body is the site of health and illness experience, and the object of medical and health intervention. Sociologists have examined the way that our understanding of embodiment, health and illness are largely shaped by medical and public health approaches to the body. This includes a view of the body as being a biological or genetic composition, a site of risk and amenable to alteration because of the rise of a biomedical approach to health and illness where the body is primarily viewed as a physical (and fallible) entity with a particular structure and function. In this view, the role of health care workers is to fix or optimise the functioning of the body with the tools, equipment and knowledge provided primarily by medicine.

It is only in recent years that sociology has considered the importance of the body as a social phenomenon, and this has influenced the way we understand the body and health. One reason for this is that in the early growth of sociology as a discipline, theorists emphasised 'the social' and in the process disassociated themselves from structures, including the body, which were considered to be biological. There was also a distinction between the body and the mind, related to the dominant way of thinking—Cartesian dualism.

See Chapter 2

The rise of the feminist movement drew attention to the importance of understanding the ways in which bodies are interlinked with social processes. For example, using biological explanations to rationalise women's unequal participation in society was one way that medicine acted as an agent of social control. Since that time, social constructionists have examined how such knowledge about bodies and body practices is shaped by prevailing social, historical and cultural factors, giving rise to an understanding of the body as more than a biological entity. Social constructionists argue that we can only understand the body with 'reference to social understandings of what the body is supposed to be and how it should behave' (Gray, 2006: 64).

The body and disability

If we accept that the way we view others' bodies and experience our own body is the result of social and cultural processes, the disabled body presents a range of issues that challenge ideas about the social construction of normality. The challenges start with the definition of disability. The most common way of defining disability relates to a deficit in the capacity to function in our society. For example, the World Health Organization (1976) defines disability as 'any restriction or lack (resulting from an impairment) of ability to perform an activity in the manner or within the range considered normal for a human being'. However, such definitions are criticised because they fail to acknowledge adequately the extent to which aids, equipment, technology and medication can reduce the disabling effects of an impairment and thus allow people to perform the tasks of daily living. The focus on 'normality' marks out people with disabilities as 'abnormal' (Barry & Yuill, 2002: 106), suggesting that it is the person that is problematic, rather than the broader social setting that defines normality. A different approach argues that disability is better defined as 'the loss or limitation of opportunities that prevent people who have impairments from taking part in the normal life of the community on an equal level with others due to physical and social barriers' (Finkelstein & French in Barry & Yuill, 2002: 107). Thus, disability becomes a measure of the disadvantage people with disabilities face in the society in which they move rather than a personal attribute. This shifts the focus of disability from an impaired individual towards social processes that create disabling conditions.

Our understanding of disability is also inextricably shaped by the qualities we value in 'normal healthy bodies'. For example, in a society that places high value on bodily control, 'unruly bodies which fail to do their owner's bidding may release powerful messages that affect the presentation of ourselves as morally competent social actors' (Pinder, 1995: 610). This may be evident through being 'out of harmony' with the 'rhythms and textures' of everyday life—for example, being unable to keep up with the pace of walking, or even of conversation, may be a marker of difference. The body becomes 'conspicuous' and separated from the qualities of the person rather than a 'taken for granted' absent presence. The disabled body may also be subjected to what Lupton (2005: 202) terms the 'averted gaze'—being viewed as invisible, thus separated from the 'normal healthy body' in practice as well as in definition.

Question for reflection

How would you define a normal, healthy body?

Approaching the body in contemporary society

As the example of disability shows, definitions of 'normal healthy bodies' are not always as clear-cut as they might appear. In the following section, we will explore some of the ways that sociologists have conceptualised approaches to the body in contemporary society. This is particularly important when we consider the role of public health activities in our lives. Public health policies and interventions are focused on groups and populations of people rather than individuals. Activities range from sanitation and environmental controls, education and surveillance, to the control of diseases that are designated as population based—for example, lifestyle diseases. Originally concerned with stopping the spread of infectious diseases through the provision of basic infrastructure, such as clean water, sewerage and quarantine measures, public health has also historically been aligned with a social view of health, promoting, for example, the provision of housing and safe working conditions as important points of intervention in improving the health of populations. The current approach to public health is known as the 'new public health'—this approach to public health recognises the interplay between individuals and their environment, and where the old public health focused on improvements in physical infrastructure, the new public health extends this to individuals and their capacity to undertake actions to avoid ill health (Baum, 2002). Thus, whereas in the old public health, bodies tended to be viewed as sources of contamination, in the new public health, bodies are often viewed as potential 'risk factors', the causes of which arise from a complex interplay of individual action, social environment and social structure.

The body as a site for regulation

In *The Birth of the Clinic*, Michel Foucault (1973) traces the rise of medicine, and the introduction of hospitals, arguing that the introduction of the hospital and the development of technologies gave medicine sight and speech through which to construct or produce bodies in a significantly new way. The technologies of medicine that apparently rendered the internal workings of the body visible to medical experts, along with knowledge and language to diagnose and therefore to define bodies as subjects, ascribed an extraordinary power to the medical profession. So we became reliant on medicine to 'show and tell' us what is happening in our bodies. In *Discipline and Punish* (1977), Foucault also talks about the emergence of institutions, such as prisons, schools and hospitals that create an environment for the management, regulation and surveillance of bodies.

Foucault has also contributed to our ideas about the body in contemporary society through the use of the concept of the panopticon and ideas about 'technologies of the self' and the creation of 'docile bodies'. The panopticon is based on the model for a prison developed by Jeremy Bentham, the originator of utilitarianism. The design involves a circular building with all the cells facing inwards and visible from a central tower in which the prison guards are located. The prisoners cannot see the guards from their cells, although they know they are present and may or may not be watching them at any time. The guards have a full 360-degree view from their watch tower, and their power clearly resides in the fact that the prisoners do not know whether they are actually being watched at any one time. As a result, the prisoners monitor their own behaviour constantly, in case they are being watched. They become their own regulators, controlling or disciplining their bodies themselves or developing 'technologies of the self' in the belief that they are constantly under surveillance. As Foucault (1980: 155) writes: 'There is no need for arms, physical violence, material constraints. Just a gaze. An inspecting gaze which each individual under its weight will end by interiorizing to the point that he [sic] is his own overseer, each individual thus exercising this surveillance over and against himself.'

This conceptual approach is useful in analysing the ways that the contemporary discourses of public health and health promotion operate to produce a 'docile' population. The linking of particular behaviours with an underlying value judgment about 'goodness' or responsibility, results in moral regulation of populations. In other words, these discourses indicate social norms and values, and imbue them with a moral imperative: the virtue of 'wellness', and health as a secular means to salvation (Conrad, 1994). Thus we engage in practices that 'discipline' our body regarding weight, exercise, smoking or drinking, safe sex, not only because we believe the health benefits, but also because of the values that are attached to having a 'disciplined body'. The capacity to regulate one's body and to 'engage in strategies of self-discipline' is important in contemporary Western society (Lupton, 2005: 202–3). Signs that our body is not disciplined, particularly visible signs such as overweight, carry social meanings of being 'out of control' in a world where control is highly valued. Such an emphasis on the creation of the disciplined and 'docile' body is criticised because it means that the focus is on individual behaviours and appearances to the exclusion of social and environmental factors important in shaping health and health outcomes. As Shilling (1993: 5) says, 'at a time when our health is threatened increasingly by *global* dangers, we are exhorted ever more to take *individual* responsibility for our bodies by engaging in strict self-care regimes'. This form of looking inward 'prevents substantive criticism of social behaviours' (Spitzack, 1992: 65).

Questions for reflection

In what ways do you 'discipline' your own body? Why?

The body as an ongoing project of the self

Contemporary ideas about individualism and the importance of exercising control lead us to understand our bodies as an 'ongoing' and important project of self-care. This approach is particularly seen in discourses around lifestyle and lifestyle diseases. Understanding the broader social context assists in making sense of the idea that our body is an ongoing 'self project'. Historically, our social position and social identity were closely linked and relatively stable. We were born into a particular social setting where the expectations were fixed, particularly in relation to social class and gender. Giddens (1991) argues that this is no longer the case in contemporary society. Contemporary society is characterised by a loosening of the social bonds through which we gained our identity, and our lives are now much less stable and much more risky. He sees this as providing the conditions through which we can create our own identity, by continually reflecting on who we are and who we wish to become in the light of increased exposure to knowledge and experiences. Therefore, we have a responsibility for shaping our own 'life story', and enter a process of 'becoming' who we want to be. Indeed such a biography may be made and remade. As part of this identity construction, 'body projects are attempts to construct and maintain a coherent and viable sense of self-identity through attention to the body, particularly the body's surface' (Gill et al., 2005: 40). The body is represented as a site over which we are able to exercise control, both through the opportunities we have regarding lifestyle, and also through the medical knowledge and technological advances that enable body alteration. Thus the body 'is seen as an entity which is in the process of becoming; a project which should be worked at and accomplished as part of an individual's self identity' (Shilling, 1993: 5).

Coexisting with this view of the body as a project, is the idea that the body is also a 'commodity'—that is, it is viewed as an item of economic value. The idea can be applied at a number of levels. For example, consider contemporary debates about the idea of bodies for 'spare parts' in the form of transplants, organ donation and stem cell research.

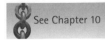 See Chapter 10

These debates raise important issues—for example, the potential exploitation of poorer people for body parts—and it is possible to see that these are not so much scientific or medical ideas, but deeply ingrained social ideas and values about such issues as exploitation, privacy and the sanctity of one's body parts. The issues are encapsulated by Scheper-Hughes (2001: 2) when she asks 'why are markets in human bodies, body parts, sexual favors, reproductive material or blood sports (like boxing) so disturbing, so hard to take?'

While some of these issues have always been debated, a globalised world has increased the possibilities in both positive and negative ways. Globalisation reflects a social, cultural and economic shift from local to global ways of thinking and acting. The effects of globalisation are evident in transnational trade, worldwide communication and transport systems. Improved communication and transport have contributed greatly to the capacity to carry out a range of practices associated with the body. Examples include telemedicine, organ donation and transplantation. Globalisation also means that the spread of disease can now be seen as a 'global problem' due, in part, to changed patterns of mobility and the creation of opportunistic, sometimes exploitative practices. An example may be the burgeoning sex trade in Third World countries, where selling one's body is a way out of poverty, but is simultaneously exploitative because the sex workers are disempowered and exposed to additional health risks. Similarly, international surrogacy arrangements are potentially opportunistic as well as exploitative.

The idea of commodification can also be applied to the ways in which we can work on our bodies to achieve desired benefits. Such benefits may not be medical necessities, but based on social values relating to appearance. A consumerist approach reinforces the idea that purchasing can remedy a range of body 'problems' (Langer, 2002: 60). Debates about cosmetic surgery reinforce the way in which we commodify the body. Such surgery holds the power to transform people into the 'idealised' body, which is constantly reproduced and reinforced. As the feminist writer Susan Bordo (1993) points out, while many advocates of cosmetic surgery maintain this provides women (and increasingly men) with a choice about their bodies and is therefore empowering, the bodily ideals that are available through surgery reinforce particular social ideas and values. The norms of beauty, power and success to which women aspire (or freely choose to adopt) are the dominant cultural forms and preferences that are racially, ethnically and heterosexually inflected. Speaking of the USA in particular, Bordo (1993) says, 'this system is reflected in the sorts of surgery women request: does anyone in this culture have her nose reshaped to look more 'African', or 'Jewish' or one might add, do people have their skin colour darkened?'

Anti-ageing is also an important self project and one where ideas about the body intersect with commodification. Here, social values and medical knowledge intersect in their negative values about ageing. This intersection is successful

See Chapter 6

because ageing is constructed both as undesirable and as a disease. Further, in a society where the 'normal healthy body' is a young body, avoidance of the appearance of ageing becomes not only a socially sanctioned ideal, but also a consumerist imperative. Vincent (2006) argues that the intersection between social values and medical constructions regarding ageing can be seen through categorising the growth of anti-ageing products that are available. First, there are anti-ageing products designed to disguise the signs of ageing. These include anti-wrinkle creams, and other skincare preparations. Second, prophylactic measures are designed to stave off the onset of physical ageing and its signs. These include the promotion of exercise regimes and a focus on diet and vitamins. Third, he argues there are compensatory mechanisms that are designed to reinvigorate the 'failing' functions of an ageing body to a youthful standard. Examples include Viagra and hormone replacement therapy. Importantly, he argues the success of these measures must be understood in the 'context of a society that has come to understand body image as the key component of personal identity' (Vincent, 2006). All of these measures reinforce the ageing body as a self project and one that is attainable through consumption.

The idea of consumption can be further explored to examine both the broadness of the health market and the suitability of the body as a product in such a market. Bourdieu's ideas are useful in understanding why we succumb to such a focus on the body. He argued that such endeavours exist as part of a cultural field (where ideas, products and practices intersect). In such a field, the producers of products and information must be able to interact through, and with, the preferences of ordinary people or consumers. Smith Maguire (2002) has applied Bourdieu's work to the study of the rise of the fitness industry and the fitness consumer. Through an examination of the exponential rise in fitness publications in the past 30 years, she takes Bourdieu's notion that there must be affinities between producers and consumers. She outlines four factors that have influenced the rise of the fitness industry—first, the rise of the middle class which has the resources to participate, and which sees the body as a project to be worked on for self-improvement; second, the changing social and political environment for women that enabled them to become consumers of such products in their own right, and not as consumers on behalf of families; third, the ideas of the fitness industry are congruent with

Question for reflection

Make a list of the ways in which you can create and work on your self identity by undertaking 'body work'. How do your 'body practices' fit with the analysis provided above?

contemporary health promotion practices in shaping responsiveness for self-responsibility in health; and finally, the expansion of consumer products and services reinforces the notion of consumer choice in the area.

The body as a site of risk

The body can also be encapsulated as a site of risk. Ulrich Beck (1992) introduced the concept of the risk society in which he argued that contemporary society is characterised by the production and distribution of risks. The management and control of risks have become the defining features of social organisation for individuals and governments. Beck (1992) argues that the myriad of risks produced by technology and science are the very ones that are now problematic in a global sense, and the notion of risk and how to avoid it underpins our everyday lives.

The body as a site of risk is now so pervasive that it has entered our everyday understanding of health. Because risk is futuristic in orientation, attention to the potential of disease is just as important as one's current state of health. Consider the public health emphasis on 'risk factors'. Risk factors are those 'conditions that are thought to increase an individual's susceptibility to illness or disease' (Roach-Anleu, 2005: 188). The 'risk factor approach' is identified as being the dominant discourse in public health and, as Nettleton (1995: 237) argues, there is a 'holy trinity' of risk factors: smoking, diet and exercise.

The body is seen particularly as a site of risk when it is associated with risky practices. The example of HIV-AIDS is particularly relevant here, as it is associated with sexual transgressions in a heteronormative society and other deviant behaviour such as drug taking. It is regarded as a disease of 'lifestyles' due to the social identities of those perceived most at risk (Nettleton, 1995: 62). These groups that exist outside the norm are perceived as presenting 'a risk' to the 'general population', thus enabling discourses of morality about innocence and guilt in transmission to emerge as important (lay) explanations.

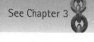
See Chapter 3

Social taboos about blood and bodily fluids, and ideas about risk are interlinked with our understanding of diseases such as HIV-AIDS, such that people with HIV 'live with the knowledge that other people are fearful of coming into contact with their blood or bodily fluids' (Chapman, 2000: 853).

Sexually transmitted infections challenge our ideas about sex, risk and bodies because of the social and moral evaluations that occur alongside the health messages about risk. This is particularly true when people are making decisions about whether to have sex with someone or not, and whether to engage in safe sex practices. This decision may be made on the basis of very little information, other than a belief of trust in one's partner or on the look of their bodies. Decisions about 'safe sex' are also embedded in social and cultural contexts that challenge the ideas of 'responsibility' and 'choice'. As Nettleton

(1995: 65) argues, messages about protecting one's body, particularly when directed at young women, 'fail to take into account the nature of power inherent in sexual encounters'. Risk knowledge, therefore, may play only a small part in the decision-making process.

Medical knowledge and technologies play an integral part in making visible and understanding the 'risky body'. Consider, for example, the case of cervical cancer. The risks are invisible to women themselves but perceived to be present. Kavanagh and Broom (1998), in analysing the experience of women who have an abnormal Pap smear, discuss the different meanings women attribute to being categorised as 'at risk' of developing cervical cancer. They find that these meanings are quite different from those of the health professionals. The experience of having a 'risky body' produces a dissociation between the body and self. The body is seen to be dangerous and threatening to the self, reinforcing a reliance on medical technologies to control and manage an inferior and inherently risky visceral body. A similar analysis can be applied to breast screening and the discourses of fear around breast cancer.

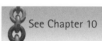 See Chapter 10

The idea of the 'liminal body' is useful for exploring the experiences of people who have a diagnosis of disease, or who are labelled as 'at risk', without any bodily signs or symptoms. This is increasingly the case in our society where technologies can enable early detection, where gene technologies can predict the likelihood of disease, and particularly where there is a focus on the body as a site of risk. All of these examples may produce a 'liminal situation: an ambiguous uncertain state wherein an individual is caught in time (and often space) between a previous status and a new status yet to be attained' (Collinson, 2005: 235). Examples include receiving a positive test result for HIV or Huntington's disease before any signs or symptoms are present. As Sachs (1995: 507) states, 'The message that you are biologically diseased without feeling ill carries the rider that disease does not necessarily proclaim its presence; a threat that does not make itself felt implies that bodily signals are not to be trusted'. Pinell (1996: 13) claims that ideas around risk have tended to 'medicalise the way each person looks at his [sic] own body'. Thus, the 'at risk' status also becomes an illness label, and increasingly people are being treated for being 'at risk' rather than for an illness itself. Kavanagh and Broom (1998) put forward the notion of 'corporeal' risk as those risks located within the body. The potentiality of disease, or liminal state, that emerges from genetic tests or other health screening tests focuses upon this idea of risk.

Questions for reflection

In what ways is your body a site of risk? What do you do to lessen these risks?

The body, public health and health practices

The ways in which we experience our bodies, together with the dominant ways that we conceptualise health and illness, are vital to our understanding of the experiences of both health and illness. As Nettleton (1995: 74) argues, 'the interpretation of symptoms will invariably be culturally specific and bound up with normative conceptions of the body'. Embedded in these experiences are the dominant ideas and values about what constitutes good health, responsibility for health and illness, and the appropriateness of health practices. Many of the body practices referred to above draw on the concept of 'lifestyle'. In contemporary public health discourses, 'lifestyle' diseases are the focus of much public health research and intervention.

Contemporary lifestyle theorists posit the claim that 'unhealthy lifestyle' is the cause of much disease in our society. Further, this explanatory framework locates the cause of such lifestyle deficit within individual control. While other broader social structural factors may be noted as descriptors of the issue, the focus of intervention thus becomes the individual. Such an approach is not entirely new in medical and public health thinking. Hansen and Easthope (2007) trace the emergence of contemporary lifestyle from historical ideas beginning with ascetic Christianity, through to moral directives aimed at restraining young people's engagement in unhealthy behaviours. Ideas about cleanliness of the body and personal hygiene, due to a fear of germs, also located responsibility at the level of the individual. With the rise of epidemiological knowledge exploring risk factors and patterns of disease, lifestyle messages associated with regular exercise, safe sex, smoking and alcohol became dominant. This is despite increasing knowledge of the social factors that also contribute to health and illness. Hansen and Easthope (2007) argue that the uncertain, anxiety-ridden conditions of modern society also lend themselves to a focus on a lifestyle that is seen to be within the control of individuals. It is in such an environment that we see health policies on nutrition, exercise, drug taking and sexual behaviour as the predominant ways of preventing and controlling disease in contemporary society. Where public health measures may once have been concerned with broader social determinants of health, a lifestyle focus individualises public health programs and interventions.

However, the new public health takes a different explanatory approach to lifestyle, arguing that lifestyle issues may be important, but that they occur within a social and cultural setting that is influential. Such an approach has the capacity to shift the emphasis in interventions from individual actions to broader community-based approaches. Hansen and Easthope (2007) also point to the importance of 'wellness nursing' as an approach that shifts the intervention from one that blames individuals for poor lifestyle to one that works with individuals to achieve better health outcomes. However, while both approaches shift the emphasis, the focus in practice remains on individuals controlling and modifying their lifestyle. Thus, ultimately bodies are individual rather than collective in their focus, raising the structure-agency debate again.

Obesity—a lifestyle disease?

Public health discourses point to obesity as a leading and preventable cause of ill health and as an urgent matter. With estimates that 9 million Australians over 18 were overweight in 2001, with 3.3 million of these in the high-risk obese group (National Obesity Taskforce, 2002), obesity is presented as an alarming epidemic. Reports about obesity point to the financial burden placed on governments and society, and the causes emphasised focus both on 'overeating' and 'underactivity'. It is generally noted that obesity is more common among lower socioeconomic or socially disadvantaged groups, higher among women in these groups, and that Aboriginal and Torres Strait Islander peoples have twice the rates of obesity as the general population.

While not wishing to detract from the health issues that may be associated with being overweight, we need to consider the ways that such an issue is constructed in contemporary Western society, in particular, how the disease is defined and treated as an individual problem, rather than an issue for society.

Consider first the ideas about being overweight as physical signs of lack of control and 'overindulgence' (Lupton, 2005), and the strong moral imperatives around containing such bodies. The roles of medicine and science are important in our understanding of how to categorise overweight. The body mass index (BMI) is a standardised measure based on population studies of the current 'ideal' measurement by which we can ascertain whether someone is overweight or not. It is argued that having the capacity to 'measure' a risk factor may in fact contribute to whether it is seen as a disease or not (Jutel, 2006). Historically, more descriptive and individual measures of overweight were used to ascertain whether a person was at risk of illness because of their weight. Jutel (2006) points to recent studies that problematise the capacity to measure overweight using the BMI as a measure. There is also criticism about whether 'overweight' in itself is a disease (Jutel, 2006). In fact, in considering the elective affinities discussed above with regard to the fitness industry, we may find a similar analysis useful when considering weight. Jutel points to the historically and culturally contingent ideas about normality and size. 'How one looks, and how close that look is to normative expectations is of

case study

➤

case study

great importance in Western society' (Jutel, 2006: 2272), and differing groups draw upon different explanations when accounting for body size (Backett-Milburn et al., 2006). However, there is little consideration about why certain groups in society are more likely to be overweight or the knowledges that may shape ideas and values about health, the body and food, other than to attribute poor eating or lifestyle habits, to the group. The dominance of the idea that 'overweight' is a 'lifestyle disease' means that it becomes difficult to look beyond the discourses to critique the knowledge base or to posit alternative ways of viewing the issue.

The 'problem' of overweight in Western societies has also emerged at a time of great social change. Consideration of the factors that shape the attractiveness and availability of energy-dense foods, and the advertising of these foods may present a different focus. Because of the pervasiveness of consumer rights and choice, what we eat and how we exercise becomes more of a problem for individuals than for governments and other social groups. The need to create supportive work environments for healthy eating and exercise occurs in a context where people are working harder and longer, where work is more likely to be contractual or casualised. Indeed, Short (2004) argues that fat is an issue of fairness, where the most disadvantaged groups in our society are more likely to be obese. Beyond describing groups at risk, there is little attention to examining the structural factors, such as level of education or income, that may contribute to predisposing a group of people to greater risk. A public health focus that emphasises the need for information and education about lifestyle individualises the problem, and can lead to victim blaming.

Questions for reflection

What are the social changes that have occurred at the same time as the rise in obesity? How might we reframe the overweight/obesity debate? How would this change the way we approach the problem of overweight in contemporary Australian society?

CONCLUSION

In this chapter, we have argued that understanding the experience of health and illness must commence with an exploration of the body in contemporary society. It is only with reference to the social processes that shape our experience of ourselves in contemporary society that we can begin to understand why people engage in particular health practices.

And the range of health practices that we engage in is vast—from bodily practices around dieting and exercise, to medical interventions such as testing and cosmetic surgery, and to altering our sense of self through the purchase of consumer products. The decisions we make about seeking medical help are inextricably linked to social ideas and processes. Similarly, consideration of 'different' bodies—such as the case of the disabled body—highlights how the construction of the 'normal, healthy body' powerfully influences our understanding of ourselves and our place in society.

REVIEW QUESTIONS

1   Why is it important for nurses to understand the sociology of the body?
2   Is the idea of the 'docile body' a fruitful way of improving health in our society?
3   Reflect on Shilling's point that we are focusing on individual behaviours at a time when our health is threatened by global dangers. How can we incorporate broader thinking about health into our understanding of health risks?
4   Why is the 'disabled body' illustrative of the ways in which we construct normality in contemporary society?
5   Are the aesthetics of contemporary body practices compatible with achieving good health outcomes?

KEY TERMS

Commodity/commodification
Consumption
Cultural capital
Embodiment
Gender identities—femininity/masculinity
Globalisation
Heteronormative

Lifestyle
Liminal body
New public health
Panopticon/technologies of the self/
    docile bodies
Risk/risk society/risk factors
Social class—habitus

FURTHER READING

Bordo, S. 1993, *Unbearable Weight: Feminism, Western Culture and the Body*, Berkeley, University of California Press.
Conrad, P. 1994, 'Wellness as a virtue: morality and the pursuit of health', *Culture, Medicine and Psychiatry*, 18, pp. 385–401.
Foucault, M. 1973, *Birth of the Clinic: An Archaeology of Medical Perception*, London, Tavistock Publications.

Hansen, E. and Easthope, G. 2007, *Lifestyle in Medicine*, London, Routledge.

Jutel, A. 2006, 'The emergence of overweight as a disease entity: measuring up normality', *Social Science & Medicine*, 63, pp. 2268–76.

Langer, B. 2002, 'The consuming self', in Beilharz, P. and Hogan, T. (eds), *Social Self, Global Culture: An Introduction to Sociological Ideas*, South Melbourne, Oxford University Press, pp. 55–66.

Lupton, D. 2005, 'The body, medicine and society', in Germov, J. (ed.), *Second Opinion: An Introduction to Health Sociology*, Oxford University Press, South Melbourne, pp. 195–207.

Petersen, A. and Lupton, D. (eds) 1996, *The New Public Health: Health and Self in the Age of Risk*, St Leonards, Allen & Unwin.

Shilling, C. 1993, *The Body and Social Theory*, Sage Publications, London.

Chapter 9

The Illness Experience: Chronic Illness

Introduction

Julia's mum tells stories about patients coming into hospital, getting fixed and then going home well again. A major difference between health care needs 20 years ago and health care needs today is the prevalence of chronic illness. This means that patients are more likely to have repeat admissions to hospital for the same illness, for which they may never be completely cured. As a nurse, Julia will benefit from an understanding of the social implications of chronic diseases and the reshaping of health care services that occurs in response to these health needs.

This chapter focuses our attention more closely on illness experiences that are designated as 'chronic'. Chronic illness involves a disruption of the normal taken-for-granted routines of everyday life. It impacts on our social functioning, affecting identity and our sense of self. We start by exploring how chronic illness is defined before examining the contribution of sociology to understanding the experience of chronic illness. Ideas of biographical disruption and narrative understandings inform the way that people respond to chronic illness. That some chronic illnesses may be more socially accepted than others is highlighted when we look at the concept of stigma. This chapter concludes with a brief case study of mental illness.

Objectives

After reading this chapter, you should be able to:

■ understand the significance of chronic illness in the patterns of disease in contemporary Australian society
■ discuss the importance of chronic illness on individual identity
■ critically analyse how chronic illness impacts on the lives of those affected
■ understand some of the social implications of chronic illness and disabilities for the provision of health care.

Chronic illnesses are those illnesses and diseases that are long-lasting, generally longer than six months. They can comprise both communicable (infectious) and non-communicable diseases. The high prevalence of chronic illnesses in contemporary society is indicative of changed patterns of illness. Historically, infectious diseases were the major contributors to mortality and morbidity. The experience of infectious diseases was epidemic in nature—contracting the illness quickly, reaching crisis shortly after and then either dying or surviving (see Strauss, 1981: 138). In contrast, the cause of many chronic illnesses may be multifactorial or unknown, they may emerge over a period of time, with progressive deterioration, and medical responses may focus on alleviating symptoms in the absence of cure. Short et al. (1993: 90) have described chronic illnesses as 'slow, insidious in onset, long-term in duration, and handicapping in their effects'. The Chronic Illness Alliance (2006) provides this definition of chronic illness:

> An illness that is permanent or lasts a long time. It may get slowly worse over time. It may lead to death, or it may finally go away. It may cause permanent changes to the body. It will certainly affect the person's quality of life.

Chronic health conditions range in degree from the mild, and easily relieved, to those that are more debilitating and incurable. Around three-quarters of the population report having one or more long-term health conditions. Sight conditions are the most common long-term conditions reported. Other commonly reported long-term illnesses include arthritis, hay fever, asthma and hypertension (Australian Institute of Health and Welfare, 2006). The Australian Institute of Health and Welfare claims that the highest levels of mortality and morbidity associated with chronic illness can be attributed to illnesses such as:

- Coronary heart disease
- Stroke
- Depression
- Diabetes
- Osteo and rheumatoid arthritis
- Chronic obstructive pulmonary disease (COPD). (Australian Institute of Health and Welfare, 2002)

However, defining chronic illness is not as clear-cut as is suggested above. Research by the Chronic Illness Alliance (Carter et al., 2002) demonstrates the impact of language on both the definitions used, and the responses to, chronic illness. Language is important in shaping health care provider, community and consumer responses to chronic illness. While doctors may use the word 'chronic' simply to denote a characteristic of time, the effect of labelling an illness as chronic can have negative connotations—for example, it may take away the possibility of recovery. Participants in Carter et al.'s (2002) research highlight the ambiguity and inconsistency in defining chronic illness by posing questions such as:

- Is there a difference between chronic and terminal?
- Does an illness need to accord with a degree of debilitation to be classified as a chronic illness?
- If an illness is well controlled, does it fit the definition of chronic?
- Should the definition relate only to the length of time one has the illness or should it relate to the complexity of the illness experience?

These questions become more problematic when we consider the wide range of conditions that are considered chronic. For example, one category of diseases that now comes under the umbrella term 'chronic' includes those diseases that would once have been regarded as terminal—for example, many cancers, HIV-AIDS and cystic fibrosis. There are also conditions for which the diagnosis is contested—that is, experts disagree about whether the illness exists or not. Examples include chronic fatigue syndrome, occupational overuse syndrome and even attention deficit (hyperactivity) disorder. And there are conditions such as lower back pain that are chronic in their effect, but may be difficult to diagnose. Added to the complexity for sufferers of these 'contested conditions' is the need for medical legitimacy of their condition in order to receive appropriate care and other support.

Another layer of complexity is added when we consider people who have received a diagnosis but who are not yet ill. As discussed in the previous chapter, people with an early diagnosis of, for example, HIV-AIDS, multiple sclerosis or Huntington's disease may be in what is known as a 'liminal' state—this is a state where one is in transition, in between two states of being. The diagnosis of a chronic illness in this case brings with it the inevitability of becoming chronically ill or disabled in the future, even when a person is apparently healthy in the present.

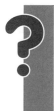

Questions for reflection

Make a list of the conditions that spring to mind when you think of chronic illness. Do they have characteristics in common, other than being long-lasting? How would you define chronic illness?

Chronic illness, biomedicine and the social

Chronic illness represents a challenge to orthodox medicine. The assumptions that underpin a biomedical approach are problematic when we consider the range of illnesses now classified as chronic, the varying trajectory that illnesses may take (there is no clear pathway from diagnosis through treatment and to cure) and the inability of biomedicine to effect a cure. The uncertainty of symptoms and diagnosis of many chronic illnesses is also challenging.

 See Chapter 2

Many symptoms are not observable or directly linked to a 'disease process'— consider chronic fatigue syndrome, attention deficit disorder and occupational overuse syndrome. The poor fit between the reporting of symptoms, their severity and the ways that doctors can test for them means that medicine's generally acknowledged expertise and authority is threatened (May et al., 2004). In the absence of definitive tests that will prove or disprove the existence of disease, 'the doctor is almost completely limited to the patient's description of symptoms' (Hyden & Sachs, 1998: 181). Notwithstanding this, doctors remain important as gatekeepers in the process of diagnosing chronic illnesses. In cases where there is considerable uncertainty about the illness, patients may need to negotiate their way through the process of diagnosis, trying to fit their description of symptoms within the biomedical framework used by the doctor in order to gain recognition of their suffering (Hyden & Sachs, 1998; Werner & Maltrud, 2003). To fit within such a framework of illness, there is a need to make the symptoms socially visible, real and physical.

Diagnosis is very important, not only because it may enable treatment, but also because it signals to the person, the wider community and other health professionals that the suffering and symptoms are legitimate. Legitimation confers a level of certainty, particularly where patients are searching for answers to unexplained symptoms; it confirms that the illness is real, that people are not malingering; and provides patients with the possibility of having their illness taken into account when they are unable to meet their social obligations (for example, work and study). Fitting many chronic illnesses into a framework defined by biomedical criteria poses difficulties for contested or medically unexplainable illnesses. In these circumstances, the doctor–patient interaction becomes important in validating the disease, ameliorating the symptoms and opening up possibilities for cure. Carter et al. (2002) argue that the medical management of chronic illness is vital to a good relationship between patient and practitioner. Their research found that people with chronic illnesses felt that their doctors were very frustrated because their illness is not curable and sometimes not treatable. Participants discussed how with each new medical encounter, they were required to 'tell their story' endlessly, thus they were loathe to change doctors because this would require them to 'train another doctor'. People with chronic illnesses thus develop a body of expert knowledge that may challenge medical authority.

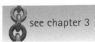
see chapter 3

Carter et al. (2002) discuss a range of social impacts experienced by people with chronic illnesses. These include the lack of community understanding of the difficulties that are experienced by people trying to fulfil the multiple roles they have to undertake to function in society. Other social impacts include the inability to work, the need for support, and poverty and isolation. As a result, people with chronic illnesses report issues of discrimination and a lack of understanding of their illnesses in both the broader social settings and in health care settings. They describe the need to meet social expectations and to 'look normal'; in some cases they are told that they 'don't look ill' and should 'try harder' to get better (Carter et al., 2002).

Participants in Carter et al.'s (2002) research also discussed the importance of being independent, but that aspiring to be independent is often a burden in itself. The recognition of limitations is difficult. What we can observe is that these responses to illness are formed in part by our social milieu. For example, consider the strong values placed on independence and control in our society; the value of appearing normal; the emphasis on wellness; the moral overtones of many health and illness issues; and the ideas around 'coping'. Gregory (2005) notes the tension between 'living a normal life' and 'following medical advice', and that 'normality' for most people does not include the lived experience of a chronic illness.

Question for reflection

What social factors do you think health workers should take into account when working with people with chronic illnesses?

Sociological approaches to chronic illness

The experience of chronic illness also challenges our taken-for-granted assumptions about the body. While it may seem that individual bodies are biological structures that are not a part of sociology, take a moment to consider how your body is part of the broader representation of who you are at any particular time. So it is for chronic illness. Our bodies are fundamental to our experiences of health and of illness. However, it is often only when our body 'lets us down' that the body as an important site of social interaction becomes

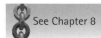
See Chapter 8

prominent. 'The body, which in many social situations is a taken for granted aspect of the person, ceases to be taken for granted once it malfunctions and becomes more prominent in the consciousness of self and others' (Kelly & Field, 1996: 248). People who experience chronic pain, for example, have heightened awareness of their bodies, but may seek to separate their sense of self from the painful body part (Osborn & Smith, 2006), seeing it as 'not part of them'. In other illnesses, the body may become a source of embarrassment, particularly when the body produces unacceptable odours or fluids. The coughing of people with COPD often results in the production of sputum, a bodily waste historically associated with physical contamination, which provides a tangible representation of the relationship between images of unpleasant sights, bad smells, disease and danger. Conscious of the effect they have on others, people whose bodies exhibit 'disgusting' aspects may withdraw from social contact in order to contain their discrediting symptoms within the private domain.

See Chapter 1

Much of our understanding about the impact of chronic illness stems from the microperspectives in sociology, in particular symbolic interactionism. This microperspective focuses on the meanings that are attached to particular actions or events. Such meanings are constructed through interaction with others, and through the interpretation of others' actions. From this perspective, sociologists have explored the ways in which identity is the product of interaction between people, and hence how chronic illness disrupts the sense of self and leads to the negotiation of new social and personal identities. There are two differing but complementary strands of sociological work that can assist in understanding individual responses to chronic illness. The first is the idea of 'biographical disruption' and the second is 'illness narratives'.

Biographical disruption

The idea of 'biographical disruption' focuses attention on the way that chronic illness is a disruption to our expected life course and events (Bury, 1982). Corbin and Strauss (1988) have described the biographical disruption in terms of a 'rupture in the connections between an individual's biographical time, conceptions of the body and conceptions of the self'. Biographical disruption sees chronic illness as a 'turning point' in one's life, requiring a rethinking of individual identity and presentation of our self to others. The concept of biographical disruption has three key features:

1   Disruption of taken-for-granted assumptions and behaviours: at this first level, the taken-for-granted aspects of the body (mentioned above) become prominent. The focus on the body or on symptoms requires the individual to acknowledge that the assumptions of health that they carry may be disrupted.

Decisions must be made about seeking help for the signs or symptoms that they notice.

2   Disruptions to the explanatory framework for illness: individuals must then consider how and why they have become ill. In seeking to put forward an explanatory framework, a fundamental rethinking of biography and self-concept is involved. For example, individuals may make sense of their illness through a range of lay ideas (see Chapter 3) or through considering their exposure to illness-creating situations over their life.

3   Response to disruption: here individuals must consider how to mobilise their resources to adjust to facing an altered life situation. This may relate to practical resources, such as financial and family supports, but it may also involve the social and cultural meanings that are drawn on to respond to the illness.

Simon Williams (2000) points to two important factors that will impact on the response to chronic illness—consequences and significance. With regard to consequences, he points to the practical consequences for individuals and families in terms of work and family relations, in the management of symptoms or medical regimens. Significance relates to the cultural meanings about the illness. This can range from those illnesses that are viewed as 'fate' or 'bad luck', to those where individual failings or personality factors are implicated and others viewed as the result of poor genes. Thus the significance of a chronic illness will impact on the way in which an individual comes to view themselves in the face of this 'disruptive event' and, it is argued, on the way that the broader society (including the medical community) may view them.

While an important concept in terms of understanding chronic illness, the idea of 'biographical disruption' has been criticised for not considering the importance of life stage or social situation as mediating the effect of a diagnosis of chronic illness. For example, the idea of biographical disruption assumes an adult-centred onset of chronic illness, where life plans are in place, and therefore does not account for children's experience of being born with a chronic illness (e.g. cystic fibrosis). There is also an assumption that one is in good health prior to the onset of illness, and consequently chronic illness forces a re-evaluation of life plans and choices that have been made on the basis of being in good health. It assumes that the onset of chronic illness marks the point of biographical disruption, rather than other 'biographically disruptive' events leading to chronic illness. 'What for some may be a disruptive experience may, for others, be part and parcel of normal everyday life, particularly in circumstances of general hardship and adversity, illness related or otherwise' (S. Williams, 2000: 61). Thus, while not doubting that the onset of chronic illness can be a disruption to one's sense of self, it is also important to consider the meaning and context within which chronic illness occurs.

Narrative understandings

Another approach to understanding the illness experience has been through exploring the narratives that people tell about their illness. It is through narratives (the stories that we tell) that people can make sense of what is happening to them, and can construct and reconstruct their identity. Narratives thus play an important role in giving meaning to our lives. 'Narratives are the means by which we render our existence as meaningful' (Whitehead, 2006: 2237). Ezzy's work seeks to examine the shaping of identity through narratives surrounding illnesses such as HIV-AIDS. He points out that symbolic interactionists have argued that 'the self was not a fixed structure or substance, but a process' (Ezzy, 2000: 609). Thus, narratives that we construct are 'in-process' and this means that 'they are necessarily unstable and may be more open to revision by some people than others' (Ezzy, 2000: 616). Thus, it is claimed, identity construction is always in-process, that narratives work to help make sense of ourselves in the face of change, and as changes occur, our sense of self may also change. The way in which we construct our story about ourself is as important as the story itself.

Consider these three narratives about illness:

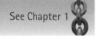
See Chapter 1

1   Restitution narrative—The plot of this narrative is that: yesterday I was healthy, today I am sick, but tomorrow I will be better. The ideas in this narrative accord with the expectations of the sick role, and with broader social ideas about illness and recovery.
2   Chaos narrative—The essence of this narrative is that: Life will never get better, no one is in control. This story may be based on one's experience, either prior social experience or the responses to illness by medicine. Any efforts to reassert predictability over one's illness or life circumstances will fail.
3   Quest narrative—In this narrative, people express acceptance of illness and seek to use this, believing that something is to be gained through the experience. Illness is thus a challenge and an impetus for change (Frank, in Whitehead, 2006).

Example: Narrative and chronic fatigue syndrome

Whitehead's (2006) research with people with chronic fatigue syndrome (CFS) reveals the ways in which narratives change. Because CFS is difficult to diagnose, and often commences with symptoms that are explained as a 'virus', participants commence their story of their illness using a 'restitution' narrative. Not getting better and the intensification of symptoms changed the narrative as people felt more out of control and scared by what was happening, and a chaos narrative emerged. People's sense of self was further challenged when their condition was not readily diagnosed and it was no longer socially acceptable to continue to adopt the sick role, even though they remained debilitated by their unexplained illness. Following diagnosis, the restitution narrative again became important as participants sought a range of treatments to alleviate their illness. Most participants also related their illness in terms of the 'quest' narrative, as they reprioritised life values, and lived within the limitations that the condition imposed, thus constructing a positive identity of living with their illness.

While Ezzy's (2000) work on narratives of people living with HIV-AIDS found similar categories to the restitution and chaos narrative, he adds a further dimension in narratives he terms 'polyphonic'. People with HIV-AIDS telling their story through polyphonic narratives talk of both hope and fear, they celebrate both life and deal with uncertainty, embracing the contradictory ways in which they make sense of their lives. 'In polyphonic tragic narratives, the uncertainty of prognosis is embraced as allowing a focus on quality of life in the present' (Ezzy, 2000: 63). While they maintain a position of agency, they also recognise that they cannot control the future. Thus Ezzy argues that polyphonic narratives allow 'a person greater flexibility to adapt to an uncertain future'.

Question for reflection

How might the ideas around biographical disruption or illness narratives be helpful to health workers working with people with chronic illness?

Stigma and chronic illness

The work of Goffman, a symbolic interactionist, is useful in understanding the ways in which people react to illness and disability. His work is an attempt to bridge people's individual situations and how they interact with broader social structures. Goffman (1963) uses the concept of stigma to refer 'to an attribute that is deeply discrediting' (Goffman, 1963: 13), and this concept helps in analysing some of the issues facing people with illnesses or disabilities. Williams claims that 'Goffman's sociology is anchored in the assumption that embarrassment is of fundamental social and moral significance' (1987: 137). It focuses around feelings of shame and embarrassment. Goffman (1963: 14) identified three types of stigma. Stigmas of the body relate to physical blemishes and deformities. Stigmas of character relate to individual deficiencies of, for example, the mind, or behaviours designated as extreme. Tribal stigma relates to social groupings such as 'race, nation, and religion'. Thus, Williams (1987: 135–6) regards stigma as 'any condition, attribute, trait, or behaviour that symbolically marks the bearer off as "culturally unacceptable" or inferior'.

Link and Phelan (2001, 2006) argue that there are five components of stigma: the first is the social process of identifying and labelling difference; second, the process of stereotyping links undesirable characteristics with the labelled person; third, social labels are used to separate 'us' from 'them'; fourth, people who are labelled suffer status loss and discrimination. The final component is the exercise of power throughout the stigmatising process, whereby power accrues to those groups who are able to label, rather than to those who are labelled.

Goffman argues that the rewards in our society are so great for being 'normal' that adaptive strategies are needed to manage and avoid stigma. Further, the notion of stigma is seen as 'spoiling' or 'disrupting' one's social identity. The likelihood of stigma may depend upon the visibility of a stigma or its obtrusiveness into everyday life. These are, of course, socially and culturally contingent. For example, a businessman in a wheelchair at a table is less likely to be stigmatised than a businessman at a meeting with severe speech impairment. Thus, people develop strategies with which to deal with stigma. Two such strategies of 'information control' that Goffman discusses are passing and covering. Passing is when the conditions surrounding the stigma are adapted to show no outward sign of abnormality and Goffman describes a wide range of techniques through which individuals seek to conceal information about a source of stigma. Similarly, Williams's (2000) research on teenagers with chronic illness examines the ways that adolescent males respond to having a chronic illness that requires medication. The disruption to masculinity felt by adolescent males is so great that they take great measures to ensure that they are seen as 'normal' in their peer groups. Characterised by secretive behaviours around the source of the stigmas, one of the prices of passing is living constantly in a state of high anxiety, as there is a myriad of ways in which efforts to pass can be revealed. The second strategy is 'covering', whereby the discredited attribute is acknowledged or obvious through processes of interaction, but there is an attempt to reduce the associated tension by making the source of the stigma less obtrusive, and therefore not the focus of attention.

The concept of stigma is important in the sociology of health and illness, because it enables an understanding of the ways that certain illness conditions constitute roles that may permanently dominate an individual's life. Using the concept of stigma enables us to explore the personal (including adaptive techniques) as well as the socially stigmatising consequences of everyday life. We can see this as a two-way process. At a social level, stigmatised people make us uncomfortable because we face the potentiality of something similar disrupting our own sense of identity. Further, stigmatised conditions threaten the boundaries of what we see as socially acceptable or desirable.

Some illnesses are stigmatised because of their association with deviant behaviour or with the perception that individuals are responsible for their illness. Again, the example of COPD is illustrative—publicly perceived as a disease resulting from smoking, sufferers are particularly susceptible to social isolation and lack of understanding. Diseases such as many sexually transmitted infections, including HIV-AIDS, are similarly stigmatised because of the judgments made about the deviant behaviour of individuals.

While a common response to ideas about stigma is that people who are stigmatised bear the brunt of discrimination and prejudice, Scambler and Hopkins (1986) argue that this is too simplistic. Their study of people with epilepsy divided the experience of stigma in two ways. 'Enacted' stigma is the experience of being stigmatised by others in society, and, they argued, that this is less prevalent than is commonly believed. However, 'felt' stigma refers to a person's view of themselves, and their feelings of shame about the possibility of enacted stigma. In this way, 'stigma-bearers share the same value system of those around them and thus experience a sense of shame' (Nettleton, 1995: 91).

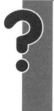

Question for reflection

Think for a moment of the types of conditions that are likely to be stigmatised. Why do you think these conditions are highly stigmatised and others are less so?

Mental Illness

case study

Dave is a 32-year-old male who works at a timber mill. He has always seen himself as a 'happy-go-lucky' kind of guy. He is married to Emma and has two sons, Harry and Blake. Dave and Emma have bought a house near Dave's work in a quiet rural town; the house is bigger than their last one, which did not have enough room for two growing boys. Their increased mortgage repayments have meant that Dave has taken on more hours at the timber mill and as a result, has less time for himself and his family. Recently, Dave and Emma have been arguing a lot because Dave is so tired when he gets home from work, as is Emma from looking after the boys all day, maintaining the household and trying to fit in her online studies in interior design. The house has been tense for weeks and Dave's relationship with his boys and Emma is rapidly declining.

At work, Dave is distracted and lacking focus. He isn't mixing well with his colleagues, who have noticed a difference in him and his work standards. He seems angry, reserved, uninspired and unmotivated, which is vastly different to his usual self. Lately, Dave's colleagues have heard him talking to himself about

case study

strange things, including suicide and how he could harm himself in the machines at the mill. This is of great concern to some of Dave's colleagues, but others make fun of him because they think he's losing his mind. None of Dave's colleagues feel as though they want to approach him about his changes in behaviour and personality; some are fearful of confronting him because they are unsure of what he might do given his recent behaviour, but others enjoy coming up with new nicknames such as 'Looney-tunes' and 'Madboy Dave'. They even liken him to a person they have seen on a supermarket advertisement on the television who is characterised as 'crazy'.

Emma has also noticed that Dave has become extremely withdrawn at home. He is not eating well and has started sleeping in the loungeroom because he is so restless at night. Often Emma finds him still sitting up and watching television at 4 am. Harry and Blake are finding Dave's absence from the home quite distressing; when Dave gets home from work they both try desperately to get his attention, which usually ends in tears, fights and shouting between everyone.

Last night when Dave got home from work, Blake and Harry were, as usual, vying for their Dad's attention. Dave feels really wound up by his sons' antics and tells them sternly that he can't cope. Emma is upset at observing her husband's behaviour and immediately starts crying. Dave grabs his keys, jumps in his car and drives to the pub where he drinks all night until closing. He sleeps in his car in the car park for the evening and somehow gets himself to work the next day.

At work, Dave's colleagues can see that he's obviously distressed and dishevelled. Some of them are taking great joy in Dave's state and continue to call him names. A few of the workers start to poke fun directly at Dave. At first he doesn't seem to even notice it—he is staring into one of the cutting machines, which he has been doing all morning. John, one of Dave's colleagues, eventually throws a piece of woodchip at Dave to try and get his attention, at which point Dave lays down on the cutting machine conveyor belt and tries to cut himself in half. He has a very blank expression on his face and says nothing when some of the workers fortunately get to him before he is able to hurt himself.

Dave is obviously in a state of despair since his life has started going downhill following a series of very stressful circumstances. In the months following the incident at the timber mill, Dave undergoes a series of assessments, and sees a psychologist and a social worker. None of his work colleagues have bothered to find out how he is and Emma and the boys are currently living at Emma's parents' house. He continues to feel isolated and depressed even though he has to take a number of prescribed antidepressant medications.

Questions

1   Identify some of the triggers that may have led to Dave's mental health issues. How are they acting as a biographic disruption? Do you think they are legitimate triggers of mental illness? Why or why not?
2   Why do you think some of Dave's colleagues were afraid to confront him about his changes in behaviour? What would you do in their situation? Why did other workers at the timber mill call Dave names?
3   Do you think people with mental illness are viewed positively or negatively in the media? Can you think of any examples?

Mental illness is surprisingly common in our society, and despite the range of conditions and the heterogenous causes and effects, the 'umbrella term' mental illness is highly stigmatised. It is estimated that more than one million Australians suffer from mental illness, with almost all of these being long-term conditions (Mathers et al., 1999). The ways in which mental illness manifests itself are seen as becoming part of that person, and thus mental illness is perceived as a 'total moral state', reflecting the sick person's total being. It often becomes a 'master-status' with existing roles, such as family and occupational, undergoing drastic reinterpretations. Schulze and Angermeyer discuss the stigma associated with schizophrenia as a 'second illness' (2003: 299). Various theorists have noted that once labelled as mentally ill, the stigma of that illness remains with the person forever—even if appearing the same as the rest of us, the person is always regarded as 'not the same'. Goffman (1963: 26) notes that 'ex mental patients, for example, are afraid to engage in sharp interchanges with a spouse or employer because of what a show of emotion might be taken as a sign of', with the effect that the mental illness label continues to provide a lens through which a person's behaviour is viewed.

The consequences of such stigma can be seen in discrimination and prejudice against people with mental illness. People with mental illness are stereotyped as dangerous. Phelan et al. (2000) note that while there has been greater public acceptance of the wide variety of mental illnesses during the past 50 years, there is a greater fear associated with serious mental illnesses, with an increase in the connection people make between psychosis and violence. One effect of such fear is 'social avoidance'—unwillingness to spend time or associate with people who are mentally ill. While there are effects at the interpersonal level, such stereotypes consolidate the social vulnerability of mentally ill people through the denial of such fundamental things as employment or safe housing.

While historically people with mental illnesses were physically separated from the community and housed in institutions, deinstitutionalisation policies from the 1980s onwards focused on community-based care and integration (Hazelton, 2004). One expectation was that the integration of people with mental illness into the community would broaden community acceptance. Richmond and Savvy (2005) argue that this has not occurred. Seeing mental illness purely as a biological disorder, they argue, increases community fear because of the perceived 'incapacity for self-control' (Richmond & Savvy, 2005: 220) when this is the dominant explanation. They also point to the role of the media in maintaining this level of fear. As a result, people with mental illness still face stigma and marginalisation even though they are located within community settings. As Hocking (2003) points out, while mental illness remains stigmatised, '*living in* the community does not mean *being part* of the community'.

CONCLUSION

This chapter has explored the range of issues associated with experiencing chronic illness. In doing so, it has encapsulated the idea that being sick is a social experience, as well as a biological one. Our identity is shaped not only by the ways we experience illness, but also by how we account for it and in the ways that others around us explain illness and its associated behaviours.

REVIEW QUESTIONS

1   Is the term 'chronic illness' now so broad that it is meaningless? How else can we describe and label the range of illnesses that are included in the term 'chronic'.
2   How can sociological knowledge contribute to health workers' understanding of chronic illness?
3   What does Williams (2000) mean when he argues that we need to 'extend the biographical focus' on explanations of the impact of chronic illness?

KEY TERMS

Biographical disruption
Chaos narrative
Chronic illness
Covering
Enacted stigma
Felt stigma
Illness narratives

Legitimation
Passing
Polyphonic narrative
Quest narrative
Restitution narrative
Social avoidance
Stigma

FURTHER READING

Australian Institute of Health and Welfare 2002, *Chronic Diseases and Associated Risk Factors in Australia, 2001*, Canberra, Australian Institute of Health and Welfare.

Bury, M. 1982, 'Chronic illness as biographical disruption', *Sociology of Health & Illness*, 4, pp. 167–82.

Carter, M., Walker, C. and Furler, J. 2002, *Developing a Shared Definition of Chronic Illness: The Implications and Benefits for General Practice. GPEP843 Final Report*, Chronic Illness Alliance/ Health Issues Centre, Victoria.

Chronic Illness Alliance 2006, 'Homepage', www.chronicillness.org.au, accessed 22 September 2006.

Corbin, J.M. and Strauss, A. 1988, *Unending Work and Care: Managing Chronic Illness at Home*, San Francisco, Jossey Bass.

Goffman, E. 1963, *Stigma*, Englewood Cliffs, Prentice Hall.

Hazelton, M. 2004, 'Mental health, citizenship and human rights', in Grbich, C. (ed.), *Health in Australia: Sociological Concepts and Issues*, Frenchs Forest, Pearson Education, pp. 200–15.

Kelly, M. and Field, D. 1996, 'Medical sociology, chronic illness and the body', *Sociology of Health & Illness*, 18, pp. 241–57.

Link, B.G. and Phelan, J.C. 2001, 'Conceptualising stigma', *Annual Review of Sociology*, 27, pp. 363–85.

Mathers, C., Vos, T. and Stevenson, C. 1999, *The Burden of Disease and Injury in Australia*, Canberra, Australian Institute of Health and Welfare.

Nettleton, S. 1995, *The Sociology of Health and Illness*, Cambridge, Polity Press.

Scambler, G. and Hopkins, A. 1986, 'Being epileptic: coming to terms with stigma', *Sociology of Health and Illness*, 8, pp. 26–43.

Short, S.D., Sharman, E. and Speedy, S. 1993, *Sociology for Nurses: An Australian Introduction*, South Melbourne, Macmillan.

Strauss, A. 1981, 'Chronic illness', in Conrad, P. and Kern, R. (eds), *The Sociology of Health and Illness: Critical Perspectives*, New York, St Martin's Press, pp. 138–49.

Chapter 10

Contemporary Debates about Health and Illness

Introduction

Our experience of health and illness is increasingly shaped by medical technologies. Some commentators argue that we are now so dependent upon technologies in health care that there has been a major shift in the use of medical knowledge and in the ways in which we understand the experience of being healthy or ill. Advances in health knowledge have undoubtedly improved the capacity to treat illness. However, what is often unacknowledged is the increased nature of uncertainty surrounding much contemporary illness, the role and scope of medical technologies in health care and the intensification of the focus upon individual attributes and behaviours as determinants of health status.

Taking a critical sociological perspective to analyse how technologies shape our experiences of health and illness requires that we explore ideas and values about technologies and the power relations that may exist in this contentious area. In this chapter, the diversity of technologies in contemporary health care provision is illustrated by examining, first, genetic technologies and then pharmaceuticals. The example of genetics highlights issues of rights and access to technologies, as well as the uncertain boundaries between health and illness. The rise of pharmaceutical technologies in the twentieth century points to the need to understand the creation and definition of illness, the importance of understanding profit motives in health care and the contested issue of regulation.

Objectives

After reading this chapter, you should be able to:

- critically evaluate the role of technologies, particularly imaging technologies, in our understanding of health and illness
- assess the advantages and disadvantages arising from new knowledge about genetics
- critically evaluate the ways in which business interests in health contribute to ideas and knowledge about health and illness.

Technologies in health

While new technologies have benefited the delivery of health care, a critical perspective examines the ways in which technological advances may be contentious. It is sometimes difficult to do this, as the idea that technological innovation saves lives is a powerful discourse in health. We live in a society in which there is a strong belief that we can, with the aid of science and technology, progress to a much better world; that we can fix problems using the truths of science and the application of technology. Such a premise assumes, therefore, that where technology is good, more is better.

Question for reflection

Make a list of contemporary health technologies, and then compare this with other people in your class. From the list you have compiled, can you define what technology is?

There is considerable debate about how best to define technology. It would not be surprising if the list you have compiled primarily related to an 'object'. As MacKenzie and Wajcman (1999) say, this 'hardware' definition is the first of three components that are important in defining a technology. Second, defining health technologies requires a consideration of how the technology refers to human activities. Health technologies ranging from the stethoscope to the X-ray are not simply pieces of hardware, they are understood in terms of the activities of the health workers using them. Third, 'technology refers to what people *know* as well as what they *do*' (MacKenzie & Wajcman, 1999: 3). Thus, it is important to include the systematic knowledge that goes hand in hand with the actual technological hardware, and to acknowledge that 'ways of knowing' are fundamental to the defining characteristics of technology. For example, the hardware that we call a mammography machine has two sets of knowledge that inform its use—it can be used as a diagnostic tool when there are signs or symptoms that need to be investigated, or as a screening device used on healthy women without symptoms. The machine is the same in both cases, but the knowledge base of the differing uses is fundamentally different. Sociologists argue that social processes are embedded within technologies that shape their use and value. Collyer (2004: 48) illustrates this definition with the example of scalpels and lasers as tools, which are employed in the process of cosmetic surgery—a contentious application of health technology, with social values and meaning attached. As Collyer (2004: 48) has stated, 'the concept of technology has come to refer not only to a machine or a tool, but also the way in which machines or tools work'.

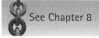
See Chapter 8

Lowe (1989) says because technology is the practical craft of solving particular problems, we often implement technologies without waiting for complete scientific understanding, proceeding instead with the knowledge that is available at the time. Health provides a good example of an area where the absence of evaluative work on many new innovations means that the knowledge base from which some new technologies are launched is very small. Thus the social and political dimensions of new health care technology must be examined. The adoption and application of technology is, as Lowe (1989) says, an intensely political activity. While there are often attempts to place it in the hands of technocrats who will provide wise guidance based on their technological expertise, we also need to recognise that social and political values remain important in determining which technologies are supported. McKinlay (1981) argued that technologies have 'careers' that are as much about the support they receive from influential players as the efficacy of the technology itself. Attachment to particular technologies throughout the stages of their career can become so strong that even when scientific evidence indicates that technologies are ineffectual, or worse, harmful, such evidence is likely to be strongly resisted by the medical community.

An example of this phenomenon is electronic foetal monitoring, which is the practice of monitoring the heartbeat of babies during labour, either by attaching an electrode to the baby's scalp or by strapping a device around the mother's abdomen. Electronic foetal monitoring has not been shown to provide any improvement in morbidity or mortality for mothers or babies (Bassett et al., 2000: 530). Studies have shown that while the monitor itself is reliable in providing data about foetal heart rates, *interpretation* of this data varies to the extent that 50 per cent of readings are false-positive—that is, they wrongly indicate problems that result in Caesarean section and other labour interventions, technologies that are also associated with an array of iatrogenic outcomes for mothers and newborns (Bassett et al., 2000: 530). The electronic foetal monitor provides an example of McKinlay's argument about the persistence of some technological practices regardless of their efficacy, but it also demonstrates the ways in which social processes mediate the ways technologies are implemented.

Questions for reflection

What kind of factors might influence the interpretation of electronic foetal monitoring data? Are these factors social or biological? What might account for the continued use of electronic foetal monitoring despite evidence that it is not a safe or effective technology? Are these reasons social or biological?

The social construction of technology

Most of us have been exposed, particularly through the media, to the idea of technologies being invented and emerging as fully informed aids to the future. Language such as 'technological breakthrough' presents us with a picture of technologies emerging independently of social and political forces. This kind of thinking is a form of 'technological determinism' and does not account for the choices that a society may make about investing in particular technologies, or ignoring others. Technological determinism does not explain why societies in the past did not make use of the technologies they had at their disposal. Or why, in the present, many inventions fail to become innovations, and many innovations are never widely adopted. Similarly, it is widely believed that economic forces drive the technologies that are adopted. While it is important to consider who invests in technologies and why, an economically determinist view assumes that we will end up with the technologies that are the most economically viable. Again, such a view denies the importance of social ideas and values in shaping the technologies that are adopted.

A social constructionist perspective takes the view that while the imperatives of economics and technology may appear to be important forces in technological change, they are in fact shaped by social priorities and values. This is important when we consider that society is characterised by a conflict of interests and values but more importantly by great inequalities of decision-making power among the individuals, groups and institutions that make up society. Therefore it would not be surprising if the technologies developed and adopted by society reflect the interest and values of the more powerful and influential members of society.

Collyer (1999: 220–1) illustrates this social construction perspective with the example of the cochlear implant. The cochlear implant is an aid to communication for deaf people. It is a surgically implanted device that uses electrical pulses to stimulate the nerves in the inner ear, thus enabling its wearer to interpret the signals that are received. However, as Collyer points out, the need for this technology emerged in a social context where deaf people are disadvantaged in social interaction because of the high value placed on aural interaction. Further, the identification of deafness as a medical problem, rather than as a sign of cultural difference, means that our society prioritises the need for a cure. Social settings where other forms of communication are the norm may not prioritise this technology in the same way that our society has. Further, Collyer argues that defining the problem of deafness as a medical problem highlights the way that such issues are individualised. 'Inequalities of power mean that deafness is defined as an individual problem requiring adaption of the *individual to society*, rather than a *social problem* requiring the modification of social practices to suit individual needs' (Collyer, 1999: 221).

 See Chapter 8

Therefore, it is argued that technology cannot be value-neutral: technology is not simply an object, which can be used for either positive or negative purposes. Rather, ideas, values and social structures are embedded within the very design of technology, and these influence and guide the way the technology will be used and the effect it will have on social life.

The expression 'technological imperative' describes the way that some cultures strongly encourage the use of a technology just because it is available. Gelijns and Rosenberg (1994: 34) explain that in the USA, medical technology is used at a much higher rate than in other countries, and that these differences cannot be accounted for by either the availability of technology or by patterns or incidence of illness. Some have argued that this culture of high-technology medicine is encouraged by a health care system that insulates individual physicians from the financial costs associated with the use of technologies (Gelijns & Rosenberg, 1994: 34). Others have suggested that the professional prestige associated with the mastery of complex machines and procedures, along with a more widespread community approval for a 'pulling-out-all-stops' approach to medicine, have combined to instil an affinity for technology among medical students (Gelijns & Rosenberg, 1994: 34). Such an imperative may modify the uses of the technology, and may expand the indications for which the technology is said to be beneficial, one example being ultrasound screening in pregnancy.

We must also consider the role that economics plays in use of technologies. 'The technological imperative is often an economic imperative with technology as the tool. What technologies are implemented and how they are implemented relates to questions of power and social control' (Willis, 1998: 172). It is difficult to withdraw a technology once it is implemented, not only because of medical and consumer expectations, but also because high technology in health requires an infrastructure (often specialised buildings as well as specialised staff), which makes withdrawal difficult. Heavy investment in technology thus shapes the technological imperative. This has been emphasised in financial arrangements through which doctors are strongly encouraged to make the most use of a technological resource for which a particular hospital may have paid millions of dollars (Gelijns & Rosenberg, 1994: 34).

There is also controversy about the extent to which technologies alter the course of the illness and treatment. Various analyses have also indicated that there may be little difference in treatment outcomes when a very invasive high technology is used compared with less invasive methods. One particular case that has occasioned attention is intensive care and coronary care units (CCUs), and the sort of treatment that is available. For example, Waitzkin (1979) argued that there is no consistent advantage of CCUs over non-intensive ward care or simple rest at home, claiming that the proliferation of CCUs was embedded in a system that was profit driven, rather than being driven by sound evidence of efficacy.

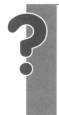

Question for reflection

Consider the following technologies—reproductive technologies; whole body scanning; cosmetic surgical techniques. What are the social ideas and values that impact on their acceptance?

Technology and the diagnostic process

One area where there has been a proliferation of technology has been in diagnosis, and this is clearly evident in our interactions with the medical profession. The array of technologies includes very basic equipment such as the stethoscope and ophthalmoscope to more sophisticated machines such as X-rays and ultrasounds, and further to more complex computerised technology such as computed tomography (CT) scanners and magnetic resonance imaging (MRI). These machines cost millions of dollars and it is argued that although they have sharpened diagnostic methods, there has not been a comparable increase in the capacity to treat or cure (Webster, 2002). The popular emphasis on visual images being able to produce certainty in diagnosis is also critiqued, particularly as clinicians draw upon a range of techniques in the diagnostic process. For example, Taylor (1979) identified the processes that are routinely involved in diagnostic medicine: taking a medical history (hearing the person's own account of the problem), which is an interactive process; an examination of the problem by the doctor; and laboratory investigations (e.g. X-ray, ultrasound, ECG, scans). Taylor argues that despite the increasing tendency to order laboratory tests, the main contributor to diagnosis is the medical history. More recently, research by Joyce (2005) on doctors' use of MRI in diagnosis points to the importance of clinical examination as well as patient history in order to 'sort out which information in an MRI image is relevant' (2005: 452). This points to the value of a good history and puts the contribution of technology in diagnosis into perspective.

Another aspect of the proliferation of diagnostic technology is the potential for overservicing. The increase in pathology and radiology testing is claimed to be second only to pharmaceuticals when measured as a cost in the health care budget (Hammett & Harris, 2002). Further, the range of reasons provided for this growth relates not only to clinical indications, but also to institutional imperatives, and social reasons, such as reassurance, that create a climate that facilitates the ordering of tests (see also Daly & McDonald, 1997). Institutional imperatives include the practice of 'defensive medicine' due to medico-legal concerns, fear of censure by one's peers and pressures to 'fast track' patients through the system. As well as increasing the costs associated with health care, there may also be adverse health effects as a result of 'overinvestigation', such as the anxiety from false positives and exposure to radiation. Hammett and Harris (2002) claim that as the number of unnecessary tests increase, so too does the possibility of a 'false-positive' test result, with exposure to possible unwarranted treatment. There is also increased potential for iatrogenic effects of illness—for example, tests such as kidney biopsy and coronary arteriography carry with them risks of side effects or adverse events.

See Chapter 2

One of the areas of growth in diagnostic technology has been in imaging technologies. These are technologies that are used to give clearer images of various parts of the body. Commencing with X-rays in 1896, there is now a wide range of imaging technologies: CT scans, positron emission tomography (PET) scans, MRI and full body scans. In fields such as cardiology, electrocardiograms (ECGs) provide images to assist in a diagnosis. However, while such technologies can assist with diagnosis where there is a clear deviation from the normal, one of the paradoxes of these technologies is that they may increase uncertainty as more and more vivid detail of the body is revealed, and it becomes unclear what in fact may constitute an abnormality. For example, with regard to cardiac imaging, Daly and McDonald (1997: 1047) state, 'While medical discourse has, for 150 years, emphasised the need for technical certainty in diagnosis, the intraprofessional discourse of diagnosis has been about how best to give meaning to the image. Technological "advance" notwithstanding, it has been impossible to draw an exact line between structurally sound and diseased hearts'. Similarly, MRIs do not produce an unmediated and truthful image of the body that conveys certain information about disease—choices made about the size of each section image, the array of artefacts that may appear on the image, and thus, the necessity for interpretation of the images produced may all shape the diagnostic process (Joyce, 2005). Further, Joyce (2005: 449) claims that this work is a 'socially situated activity'—where through a process of interaction, those working in the field develop a 'professional vision' or way of viewing the images and determining how to interpret them, thus challenging the belief that such images are objective, visual 'truths' that exist independently of interpretation and clinician knowledge.

An array of technologies is used to detect diseases in the early stages of their development, often before the person has experienced any symptoms of disease or illness—for example, screening mammography for breast cancer and colonoscopy for bowel cancer. Such screening also carries the potential for harm from the procedure itself (ranging from discomfort to actual potential for injury) as well as the emotional distress (anxiety, embarrassment) that may occur. For example, women who undergo screening mammography are exposed to X-rays and it is conceded that the screening of large numbers of women in this way will inevitably lead to some cases of breast cancer—iatrogenic-radiation-induced. For these women, the risk of potentially inducing cancer in an otherwise healthy breast is outweighed by the risk of potentially allowing cancer to be undetected. From this example, we can see how subjective notions of risk might shape attitudes towards breast screening and decisions about undergoing a mammography. The trust we place in technology to see inside the body and to provide reassurance in the absence of symptoms is a key determining factor in the choice to be screened (Willis & Baxter, 2003).

Reliance on imaging technologies has also seized the public's imagination with the popularisation of full body scans, advertising for which is directed at consumers in order to gain a 'full picture of their health'. This example highlights the ways in which increasingly healthy people are being targeted for testing, in the absence of any signs or symptoms. Critics argue that the value of reassurance is promoted above any clinical indication or benefit of the test. Not only does this place a drain on health resources, but also such tests may provide a 'false-positive' result, indicating the potential of disease where none exists, or a 'false-negative' result, indicating that all is well when it is not. As stated before, a false-positive result may expose people to increased medical intervention. Reliance on such tests reinforces the message that illness is an individual issue located solely in our biological or genetic make-up, thus further detracting from other social and political conditions that may contribute to disease causation.

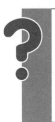

Question for reflection

What do you think are the advantages and disadvantages of using diagnostic technologies to detect diseases in otherwise healthy, asymptomatic people (e.g. mammography, colonoscopy, full body scan)?

Genetic technologies

The mapping of the human genome and the associated benefits in the early detection and application of 'gene therapy' herald the promise of a world where good health is assured. This technologically determinist perspective focuses on the ways that technology can create a better and healthier world. Alternative views of human gene therapy highlight some of the social issues and the ways in which the project is socially and politically shaped. Understanding the focus on genetics in biomedicine requires that we explore the factors that influence the ways that we explain the causes of health and illness. These explanatory frameworks in turn shape the choices that are made in relation to resourcing particular problems and their solutions. Willis (1995), in particular, draws our attention to issues of resource allocation as well as the way in which a genetically constructed view of 'normality' detracts attention from socially constructed inequities. Similarly, Lippman (1992) argues that the predominance of genetic research reinforces dominant biomedical and individual perceptions of health and illness in which scientific knowledge is seen as a major contributor to progress, downplaying the way in which health and illness are socially constructed.

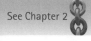

See Chapter 2

Peter Conrad argues that the public ideas about genetic explanations accord with the dominance of the 'germ theory' encased within the biomedical model. In focusing on genetics, we make the assumption that the 'internal environment is the primary causative factor' (Conrad, 1998: 231). The close fit between genetics and germ theory is one reason that the broad ideas around genetics are so readily accepted. Thus, the emphasis in genetics tends to be upon a genetic form of biological determinism, which sees that people are the way they are because of their genes rather than the sort of society in which they live (Willis, 1998). For example, there has been continued focus on the search for genes for 'obesity' and 'alcoholism' at a time when the social and environmental factors influencing these issues are well known. It is suggested that the location of genetic solutions are important in a social context where we face increased uncertainty (what some sociological writers have coined 'high modernity' or 'risk society') because genetic explanations appear to provide concrete explanations and exude a sense of certainty that is attractive in uncertain times.

The 'new genetics', a term first coined in the early 1980s, signalled the beginning of a new enterprise, with the use of different technologies and was therefore arguably different to previous ways that genetics had been understood and utilised. It was seen as a more positive way of viewing genetics compared to the eugenic overtones arising from, in particular, the Nazi era in Germany. The focus was on the possibilities for humankind in the application of genetic knowledge. This gained momentum when researchers shifted from the classical genetics associated with specific genetic diseases, to diseases such as cancer where support came from a broader base, even though the genetic links were more obscure.

An important component of the 'new genetics', and one that has received considerable publicity, is the Human Genome Project (HGP). The HGP began in 1990 and was completed in 2003. It received substantial US Government support in partnership with other countries to:

- identify the 20,000–25,000 genes in human DNA
- determine the sequences of the 3 billion base pairs that comprise human DNA
- store this information and improve tools for data analysis
- transfer related technologies to the private sector
- address the ethical, legal and social issues (ELSI) that arise from the project.

While there has been considerable attention paid to the companies that hope to make a profit from the marketing of genetic applications, there has been less attention to the ELSI aspect of the HGP. This part of the project received 3 per cent of the funding and it is notable that the HGP is the first large scientific undertaking to address these implications. However, a major criticism has been that these concerns are only addressed within the scientific framework. That is, it has not been anticipated that these concerns could actually prevent the project going ahead, rather attention to the issues is about ameliorating them as secondary concerns, with the primary focus being on the scientific and commercial knowledge.

Private-sector involvement in genetic technologies is particularly disturbing for those concerned with equitable access to health care and those opposed to the 'commodification' of one's genetic make-up. The commercialisation of genetic diagnoses and therapies depends on the ability of people to pay for them. This raises questions such as whether the choice to use genetic technologies should be based on ability to pay, or whether genetic diagnoses and therapies should be funded by governments. The use of genetic diagnoses and therapies has been likened to 'buying advantages for one's children', akin to the capacity to purchase extra-curricular activities, such as piano lessons. It is also argued that for debilitating diseases such as cystic fibrosis, for which there already exists substantial genetic knowledge, further genetic diagnoses and therapies may not be commercially viable, or will be prohibitively expensive, given the relatively small populations that are affected (Stockdale, 1999: 582). Additionally, funds raised in order to search for a cure, or to support genetic research, do little for those currently living with the disease.

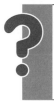

Question for reflection

Under what circumstances do you think genetic diagnosis and therapies are warranted? Give reasons for your answer.

The new predictive technologies

The new predictive technologies carry with them the prediction of future health or disease profiles based upon analysis of an individual's genetic make-up. Their target populations are those people who are presymptomatic— that is, fit and healthy individuals (over 18 years of age), prior to the presentation of any symptoms of illness. This is a rapidly expanding area of technology. Predictive genetic tests are available for over four hundred conditions and two single gene disorders are mapped daily (that is, around five hundred per year). Predictive technologies enable genetic testing of adults for what are known as autosomal dominant genetic illnesses, such as Huntington's disease. They also enable gene susceptibility testing or predispositional genetic testing for adults for conditions such as familial breast cancer, familial Alzheimer's disease, familial heart disease, familial colorectal cancers, allergic asthma, schizophrenia and bipolar disorder. Testing is also available for carrier screening for autosomal recessive conditions such as cystic fibrosis.

A sociological analysis of predictive genetic testing points to significant social issues. For example, there is potential to affect relationships because partners may be chosen on the basis of the suitability of their genetic make-up. In the 1997 film *Gattaca*, hair and skin samples replace first dates and job interviews within the new genetically constructed social order. Interestingly, the 'tagline' for the film is 'there is no gene for the human spirit', which raises the issue of whether social interests prevail over the rights of individuals.

An important issue that arises in the example above is the accessibility of genetic information. Debates about who should have access to genetic information, particularly where the information relates to the potential disease profile, rather than the actual diagnosis, are hotly contested. Knowing someone's genetic make-up may lead to genetic discrimination, whereby individuals are discriminated against because of perceived or real differences in their genetic make-up. Such information could result in the denial of access to particular services or opportunities—for example, life insurance or employment. Willis argues that this constitutes victim blaming—'focussing on individuals who are risky rather than on risky work practices or substances' (Willis, 1995: 107). In the example of employment, this is done ostensibly to protect the interests of workers; however, the effect is to screen out workers with particular genetic predispositions.

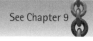
See Chapter 9
Genetic testing may result in a whole group of people being labelled the 'asymptomatically ill', that is, those who are in a 'liminal state', somewhere between health and illness.' Sociologists are interested in the individual and social consequences of this. Once someone is deemed 'asymptomatically ill', how does this shape their sense of self, their willingness to engage in activities and their interactions with others? Consider, for example, the case of Huntington's disease, a mid-life onset disease, which causes dementia and loss of motor control. Being at risk for Huntington's disease has been described as a 'time bomb' (Taylor, 2004). The ability to test people for the Huntington's disease gene has been available since the mid 1990s; however, Taylor's (2004) research revealed that few of the potentially affected people come forward for testing. Many come forward later in life, and it is thought these people may be using the test for early diagnosis of the disease rather than to establish their genetic situation. Of those who undergo genetic testing, relatively few seem to wish to use testing

for reproductive decisions or for abortions, perhaps because individuals will probably live to middle age without any symptoms. There are also issues about testing at a younger age when one's parents have not had the test, as this may convey genetic information to others as well as oneself. This raises an added complex layer to the 'right not to know' one's genetic risk (Taylor, 2004).

Question for reflection

Under what circumstances do you think genetic information about individuals should be made available to others?

Preimplantation genetic diagnosis (PGD) and embryonic stem cell research

PGD is a new genetic technology in which *in vitro* embryos are genetically screened (via cell biopsy) prior to selection and transfer to the womb (Bickerstaff et al., 2001; Braude et al., 2002). PGD can be used for sex selection (for social or medical reasons), to improve in vitro fertilisation (IVF) success rates and to screen embryos for chromosomal abnormalities and inherited genetic diseases (Robertson, 2003). It can also be used to screen embryos in order to produce a child who is a tissue match (and donor) for an existing child (Bellamy, 2005; Gavaghan, 2003) and recent indications suggest that PGD may soon be used to screen for susceptibility to adult-onset illnesses, such as cancer and Alzheimer's disease (Robertson, 2003: 213; Zeiler, 2004: 177). PGD differs from other forms of prenatal testing because it takes place prior to implantation of the embryo in the womb, thus avoiding termination of pregnancy (Cameron & Williamson, 2003). PGD has become the subject of public debate in Australia and overseas. As Robertson (2003: 213) states, 'PGD is ethically controversial because it involves the screening and likely destruction of embryos, and the selection of offspring on the basis of expected traits'.

The expression 'designer babies' is often used as a kind of media shorthand during discussions of PGD to suggest that PGD represents a threat to 'natural' conception. However, in speculating about the role of technology in the creation of 'families of the new millennium', Gilding argues that genetic engineering is likely to become so ubiquitous that the expression 'designer babies' will become passé (2002: 7).

The use of embryonic stem cells in medical research is another controversial genetic technology that has generated public discussion in Australia and overseas. Embryonic stem cell research uses 'leftover' IVF embryos, cord blood cells and cells from aborted foetuses. Embryonic stem cells are useful in medical research because they are what are known as 'undifferentiated' cells. A simple explanation of this is that they have the capacity to transform into any organism in the human body. Thus, for example, scientists can turn stem cells into breast tissue and then experiment on that tissue to see what effect particular toxins might have. Embryonic stem cell research is often described as therapeutic cloning because these cells have the capacity to regenerate themselves indefinitely. In embryonic stem cell research, embryos consisting of less than a dozen cells can be used for ongoing research into illnesses ranging from diabetes to cancer.

The idea of what an embryo might look like, contrasted with the idea of a small number of cells sitting in a Petri dish, highlights how debates about the technology might be shaped by interpretation. As David and Kirkhope (2005: 367) explain, 'the meaning of terms, and their ambiguity, is a significant factor in ethical debates, policy and practice'. These differences in interpretation, or perspective, are illustrated in debates about the so-called 'snowflake children'. These are children that are born from 'leftover' IVF embryos that have been donated to another family. The interpretative distinction between an embryo and a collection of cells mirrors the distinction between the concept of an embryo as a potential child or as a potentially life-saving resource for medical science. One side of this debate draws on the imagery of a happy, healthy baby born into a worthy family, and this contrasts with the idea of millions suffering from illnesses that might be cured by stem cell research. Both perspectives are framed by an ethical discourse that protagonists draw upon to justify and promote their position. Embryonic stem cell research was recently legalised in Australia after a divisive political and public debate (Murphy & Stafford, 2006). Media representations of this debate highlight the differences in the ways people interpret the idea of embryonic stem cell research:

See Chapter 4

> Therapeutic cloning advocates last night hailed the vote as a victory for science and hope, while opponents warned it was the first step towards a brave new world in which life is created for functional purposes and then destroyed. (Murphy & Stafford, 2006)

While most people would not deny the significant benefits that can potentially arise from genetic technologies, a sociological analysis means that we locate our understanding of the benefits and costs of such technologies within a social framework. As Willis says, 'genetic research and technologies are shaped by the sort of society in which we live. The social aspects are not merely technical details of implementation' (1995: 112). Genetic technologies involve a complex array of social, economical, ethical, scientific, technological and legal issues. Often the 'social' aspects of technology become invisible in the debates, perhaps because it is easier to label something as an ethical or legal issue. For example, concerns about whether we should allow preimplantation genetic screening technologies are clouded in legal and ethical language, with the social seemingly an 'absent presence'.

Question for reflection

Why do you think these labels, 'designer babies', 'preimplantation genetic diagnosis', 'snowflake children', might generate different responses?

Pharmaceuticals

That technologies have social and cultural meanings is apparent when we examine pharmaceuticals and their use in contemporary society. The cultural and social meanings around drug use reinforce their value in health and healing. The word drug has more than one meaning and our social knowledge must distinguish between these different meanings. 'In classic times the word had three meanings: remedy, poison, and magical charm' (Montagne, 1996: 11).

Almost 200 million prescriptions are dispensed every year in Australia. Medication is taken by 70 per cent of the overall population, and more than 90 per cent of the elderly in any two-week period (Runciman et al., 2003). The rate at which Australians are issued with subsidised Pharmaceutical Benefit Scheme (PBS) prescriptions, either through medical consultations or as hospital in-patients, creates enormous potential for adverse drug outcomes. The Australian Incident Monitoring System reports that 26 per cent of 27,000 hospital-related incidents, 36 per cent of 2000 anaesthesia-related incidents and 50 per cent of general practice incidents, were medication related (Runciman et al., 2003). However, these figures are conservative due to considerable under-reporting of adverse drug reactions.

The emergence of an industry to provide and market pharmaceuticals occurred in about the 1930s and 1940s, when it was realised that chemical knowledge developed in other industries could be applied to medicine (George & Davis, 1998: 192). At this time, new technologies were developed to produce new medicines in large quantities, and patents were granted to pharmaceutical manufacturers that gave them monopoly privileges over their innovations. The emergence of antibiotic drugs heralded a new era in biomedicine, after it was found that drugs could be targeted to specific disorders. The use of these drugs reinforced the value of drug therapy and the uncritical view of 'magic bullets' to solve all health problems. However, there is not a clear pathway from medical problem to scientific innovation and subsequent medical intervention. One way we can illustrate this is by examining the number of pharmaceuticals that have uses (and markets) for which they were not originally intended. For example, diazepam (a minor tranquilliser) was originally intended for allergic reactions. More recently, Viagra (sildenafil) was developed to relieve high blood pressure. Perhaps the most famous of these cases is the 'compound that it was hoped would clean teeth and harden the gums, as well as relieving mental and physical exhaustion. It failed dismally in the form of a medicine but succeeded beyond belief in the form of a soft drink—Coca-Cola' (George & Davis, 1998: 192).

The influence of the pharmaceutical industry on the delivery of health care is pervasive in that while not easily recognisable to the consumers of care, it significantly influences policies about health and the health care received. 'In most industrial countries, although they try to maintain a low profile, the drug manufacturers are among the most powerful political and economic pressure groups' (Melville & Johnson, 1982: 5).

Pharmaceutical use and acceptance are premised on a much more complex interplay of social factors than simply efficacy or evidence of benefit. A sociological approach to examining pharmaceuticals points to the importance of production techniques; the ideas and values in society about the acceptability of drug therapies; the alignment of pharmaceuticals with medical knowledge, thus increasing their authoritative value; and the legitimation of pharmaceuticals by doctors and by the state (through acceptance on the PBS).

A critical issue in the exploration of pharmaceutical drug use is who decides that a condition exists as an illness that must be treated. Kawachi and Conrad (1996) point to the influence of pharmaceutical companies in the determination of what constitutes high blood pressure. These companies have a vested interest in ensuring that a significant proportion of the population are outside the range categorised as 'normal'. The capacity to measure a symptom 'scientifically', and to then provide a definition of what constitutes 'normal', is a social process upon which there may be many influences. This is particularly the case when the measurement relates to 'risk factors', such as blood cholesterol, high blood pressure or bone density, rather than a disease process itself. Similarly, Coney's (1993) analysis of osteoporosis links the dairy industry, the pharmaceutical industry and medical interests, and highlights the ways in which business interests are interwoven in the marketing of health. In their book, *Selling Sickness*, Moynihan and Cassels (2005) provide several case studies of so-called 'medical conditions' that have been redefined as illness in order to create a market for pharmaceuticals. The examples they provide include 'social anxiety disorder', 'irritable bowel syndrome' and 'female sexual dysfunction', among others.

The marketing of pharmaceuticals differs from many consumer goods because prescribing doctors act as 'gatekeepers' by determining what consumers buy and what hospitals maintain in their dispensaries. Therefore marketing strategies have traditionally targeted doctors rather than the consumers themselves. To this end, the pharmaceutical industry shapes the prescribing habits of doctors, not only through the usual promotional and advertising strategies, but also primarily through the maintenance of a vast army of sales representatives throughout the world, ranging from as high as one representative for every three or four doctors in some countries, to one in eighteen in others. With the growth of generic or 'non-brand' drugs, pharmaceutical companies attempt to establish and maintain brand loyalty in order to ensure that doctors continue to prescribe their drugs instead of the cheaper generics. The doctor maintains an important role as gatekeeper, and patients are not included in this decision making, even though they must bear the cost of the drugs prescribed.

In turn, doctors are often reliant on the information provided to them by the pharmaceutical companies. Doctors are most likely to read literature produced by pharmaceutical companies in the guise of medical journals, where they receive advertising messages both in the so-called news stories (advertorials) and in the more conventional advertisements. Another point of debate is the convergence of interests in medical journal publishing. On the one hand, many journals are reliant on advertising from pharmaceutical companies as a source of income. On the other, this raises issues of promoting products/values of the advertisers. 'Our market economy rewards pharmaceutical innovation, our society demands that individuals invest in ever increasing their health status, and modern medicine is centred around "advances" and improving treatment outcomes' (Doran et al., 2006: 1517).

The role of regulatory authorities is a contested area in pharmaceutical issues. Having invested large amounts in research and development, understandably drug companies are keen to market their product as soon as possible so that they start to provide returns on the investment. The government, acting on behalf of the consumers, must ensure that pharmaceutical drugs are safe, thereby insisting on significant trial data before allowing the product to be available. In cases where pharmaceuticals are subsidised through schemes such as the PBS, it is also argued that provision of new drugs should be in the community interest—that is, that they be efficacious and economical. In their discussion of the PBS listing of Viagra, Aroni et al. (2003) claim that the interests of all the stakeholders in these debates work from values that are incommensurable. These tensions are exemplified in the recent debates about the introduction of the cervical cancer vaccine, Gardasil. During negotiations between the manufacturer of Gardasil (CSL) and the Pharmaceutical Benefits Advisory Committee (PBAC, the body that decides which drugs are subsidised by the PBS), CSL was told to resubmit its application to list Gardasil on the PBS because the price it was asking the government to pay was considered too high. Within days, a political furore followed. Stakeholders canvassed both the cost and efficacy of the new drug, and both the health minister and prime minister were forced to overrule the PBAC decision and encourage CSL to resubmit sooner rather than later—the unspoken assumption attached to this offer was that the application would be received more favourably the second time around (Stevens, 2006).

At a government level, issues of regulation may also potentially result in conflict between industrial policy and health and social protection policy frameworks. Similarly, debates about social values may be involved in issues of regulation. Consider, for example, recent debates about the 'abortion pill', RU486. The debates about regulating this drug have focused on social and moral values about abortion, as much as about the safety of the drug itself.

Questions for reflection

What does the controversy over Gardasil tell us about decisions to list drugs on the PBS? Are decisions about the PBS made on economic, scientific or social grounds?

CONCLUSION

This chapter has highlighted some contentious issues associated with the provision of health care in contemporary society. While not denying that health care provision may have changed substantially for the better through the use of technological innovations, the case studies of genetics and pharmaceuticals demonstrate the ways in which such innovations are as much about social ideas and values as they are about the efficacy of health care provision. Further, commercial interests in the health care sector are able to exert substantial influence over the ways in which we address health care problems. The alignment of genetics and pharmaceutical knowledge with the scientific paradigm means that there is less critical engagement with their promises of progress.

REVIEW QUESTIONS

Julia is surfing the Human Genome Project site and locates the sections that focus on ELSI. She questions:

1 What are the issues that are addressed as part of ELSI? How are they being addressed?

Next, Julia imagines that she has successfully undertaken IVF treatment. She has two 'leftover' embryos, but doesn't want to have any more children. She has a choice between donating them to an infertile couple, donating them to medical research, freezing them indefinitely, or allowing them to 'die' by thawing them out. She contemplates which decision she would make.

2   What decision would you make? What factors have influenced your decision? Now ask three of your classmates what they would do. Why might their decision be the same as yours? Why might it be different? Do you think any one of these choices is inherently right or inherently wrong? Who should decide what happens in this case?

Julia is also curious about the issue of pharmaceuticals and wonders:

3   To what extent do the interests of business conflict with the interests of patient care? Can this conflict be reconciled?

KEY TERMS

Asymptomatically ill/liminal state

Commodification

False-positive/false-negative

Gatekeeper

Gene therapy

Genetic discrimination

Human genome

Iatrogenic

New genetics

New predictive technologies

Normality

Preimplantation genetic diagnosis

Risk

Risk factors

Technological determinism

Technological imperative

Victim blaming

FURTHER READING

Collyer, F. 1999, 'The social production of medical technology', in Grbich, C. (ed.), *Health in Australia: Sociological Concepts and Issues* (2nd edn), Frenchs Forest, Pearson, pp. 217–37.

Collyer, F. 2004, 'Medical technology: from drugs to genetics', in Grbich, C. (ed.), *Health in Australia: Sociological Concepts and Issues* (3rd edn), Frenchs Forest, Pearson, pp. 46–72.

MacKenzie, D. and Wajcman, J. (eds) 1985, *The Social Shaping of Technology*, Milton Keynes, Open University Press.

McKinlay, J. 1981, 'From "promising report" to "standard procedure": seven stages in the career of medical innovation', *Milbank Quarterly*, 59, pp. 374–410.

Moynihan, R. and Cassels, A. 2005, *Selling Sickness: How Drug Companies are Turning Us All into Patients*, Crows Nest, Allen & Unwin.

Taylor, S.D. 2004, 'Predictive genetic test decisions for Huntington's disease: context, appraisal and new moral imperatives', *Social Science & Medicine*, 58, pp. 137–49.

Willis, E. 1998, 'The "new" genetics and the sociology of medical technology', *Journal of Sociology*, 34, pp. 170–83.

Part 4

Working in Health

In Part 4 we present various aspects of the health care system in Australia. This part applies a sociological analysis to the health care workforce, including the role and function of health professionals, as well as the interaction between them. This is achieved through a focus on the key concepts of professionalisation, legitimacy and autonomy as they apply to medicine, complementary and alternative medicine, and nursing.

The first chapter in this part, 'Health Care Systems and the Health Workforce', commences with an overview of the social organisation of health care and demonstrates how this reflects the dominant social values and beliefs in society about health and illness. The success of the medical profession in gaining professional status and state-endorsed legitimacy is discussed in depth. In contrast to this, the next chapter, 'Complementary and Alternative Medicine' explores the struggle of alternative health care practitioners to achieve legitimacy, despite increasing popularity and consumer demand. The final chapter in this section, 'Nursing in Contemporary Australia', examines how nursing roles and scope of practice have changed over time in response to professionalising strategies, and through interactions with other health professionals and clients.

Chapter 11

Health Care Systems and the Health Workforce

Introduction

The way that health care is organised in our society is a product of history, social forces and cultural values. Like other institutions, such as law and education, health care is part of our social structure. A sociological approach to understanding the health system focuses on whether the health system keeps us healthy, whether the benefits of government spending on health are fairly distributed in the community and who is authorised to provide health care.

Health care systems respond to identified social needs; however, there is a diverse range of needs that compete for priority, leading to debates over values, policy choices and resource allocation. In this way, the organisation of health care is not just a response to socially recognised needs, it must be understood in the context of the broader socio-political environment. The topics covered in this chapter include an overview of the organisation of health care, health care funding and the health care workforce. The chapter will conclude with a discussion about the challenges to the existing health care system.

Objectives

After reading this chapter, you should be able to:

- explain how the organisation of health care in Australia is a reflection of the dominant values in our society
- understand the concept of professionalisation and how it applies to health occupations
- critically analyse the dominance of the medical profession within our health care system.

The organisation of health care in Australia

Within the Australian health care system, responsibilities for health care funding and provision are divided between the federal and state governments, and there is a mix of public, non-government and private sector providers, as well as informal providers such as family, friends and community networks. The Federal Government's role is primarily in policy making and national issues such as public health, research and information management, as well as funding most medical services that occur out of hospital. The states and territories are responsible for the delivery and management of public health services and for maintaining direct relationships with most health care providers, including the regulation of health professionals. They have joint (although not equal) responsibility for the funding and provision of public hospitals, and community care for the aged and people with disabilities. The Australian Health Care Agreements determine the level of federal grants given to states and territories for public hospital funding. They are negotiated every five years. These agreements stimulate heated debate and discussion, particularly in relation to indexation, as factors such as prices and wages, demographic effects (population growth and ageing) and advances in technology place increasing pressure on the health care system. Thus, the arrangements for the organisation, funding and provision of health care in Australia are highly complex. The following discussion will demonstrate how the Australian health care system is very much a product of history and social values.

Historical context

During the early years of Australia's settlement by Europeans, three characteristics emerged that continue to influence our health care system. The first is the ability of medical practitioners to gain prominence and political influence given the variety of people that provide advice and treatments for illness and health problems. During the early 1800s, doctors were usually appointed to official positions, such as medical officers on emigrant ships or as part of the colonial public service, which also bestowed upon them power and status in society. The number of doctors was initially very small, but as they grew in number they soon began to organise themselves (for example, by forming an Australian branch of the British Medical Association) and work together to push aside competing occupations that were referred to as 'quacks' (Willis, 1989). Legislation introduced in 1838 in New South Wales required appropriately qualified doctors to be registered. It established a process of self-regulation for doctors and was a successful professionalisation strategy for medicine.

The second characteristic is the responsibility that governments have in the provision of health and welfare, which was necessary during early settlement because of Australia's role as a penal colony. As a result, Butler et al. (1999: 254) argue that the political culture in Australia includes 'a highly instrumental view of government and a traditional acceptance of the need for "big government"'. However, the government's role in the control and provision of health care has at times been challenged by the medical profession. For example, in 1946, the Australian Government sought to amend the constitution to extend its authority in health care and social welfare provision. The medical profession, through its membership of the Australian branch of the British Medical Association, strongly resisted government attempts to control health care in order to retain its independence, its fee for service preference and other interests (Belcher, 2005). Because of this resistance, the constitutional amendment extended government powers with the condition that the medical and dental professions were exempt from any form of civil conscription, such as compelling doctors to enter salaried employment or to provide services for a prescribed fee. The constitutional relationship between the government and the medical profession continues to influence (and some would argue that it constrains) the way that health care is organised because it protects the vested interests of medicine (George & Davis, 1998).

The third characteristic is the way the health care system has acute care services (hospitals) at its centre. The establishment of hospitals in the latter part of the 1800s occurred in response to the needs of the growing population and improvements in the treatment and management of diseases and illnesses, which saw hospitals change from places for the sick, poor and dying (Belcher, 2005). The increasing acceptance of hospital care can also be linked to the professionalisation strategies of nursing and medicine. In hospitals, only doctors and nurses were authorised to provide care, thus excluding other health care practitioners (George & Davis, 1998). Hospitals came to play an important role in the teaching and training of doctors and nurses. As medical care increases with complexity, so too does the size and specialisation of hospitals and the cost. In 2004–05, hospital funding accounted for more than a third of recurrent health expenditure ($29 billion). Hospitals are funded through a mix of federal and state government contributions, and these funding arrangements are under constant negotiation.

Question for reflection

What impacts do the three characteristics described above have on the contemporary health care system?

Social and political context

There are no natural limits for health-related expenditure, therefore determining the best possible arrangements for health care will often involve value judgments and include political processes because of competing interests and limited resources. Trade-offs are required between the health sector and other sectors (particularly when we consider that the health system is not the only contributor to health status); between prevention and treatment services; improving overall health and improving health inequalities; and between short-term and longer-term objectives. These trade-offs reflect social values; therefore, these decisions are often based on an underlying ideology, or beliefs and values, about the way society should be organised. Two key aspects of the social and political context that influences the organisation of health care in Australia are, first, the choice between curative and preventative health care; and, second, the extent to which health care provision should be an individual or collective responsibility.

Treatment or prevention

Services within the Australian health care system are organised in three tiers—primary, secondary and tertiary (see Table 11.1).

TABLE 11.1   Three tiers of health care

Primary health care	Entry point to health services
	Includes essential service for the care of common health problems
	Extends to illness prevention, early detection and identification, health promotion, e.g. general practice, child health services, home nursing, community development, immunisation, cervical and breast screening services
Secondary health care	Defined pathways exist for accessing these services, usually requiring referral from a doctor
	These services provide skilled and specialist care for more complex health problems, e.g. psychiatric care, gynaecological services, diabetes care, specialist physicians
Tertiary health care	These services are highly specialised and provided within hospitals, e.g. in-patient care, surgery, invasive investigations

There is considerable debate about how funding should be apportioned to these different levels of the health care system. Should the funding be allocated to illness prevention and maintaining wellness (primary health care), or should funding be spent on illness care (secondary and tertiary care)? The answer to these questions is essentially a trade-off between current health and future health.

The largest proportion of health care funding is absorbed by the tertiary sector. Modern hospitals with the latest equipment and cutting-edge techniques are viewed by some as a marker of excellence in health care. As discussed in Chapter 10, the increasing use of technology is becoming more acceptable over time, and there is evidence of a technological imperative, whereby technologies are used because they exist rather than because they are clinically necessary. The changing use of technologies is also a contributing factor.

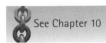 See Chapter 10

For example, complex and invasive procedures may be undertaken through the use of laparoscopy, using a lighter anaesthetic and leading to a more rapid recovery. While such changes may reduce the cost of health care, some commentators argue that they do not reduce the overall cost, as often more surgery is attempted. Many health professionals receive education and training within large teaching hospitals that have access to the latest procedures and technologies that perpetuate the use and need for these approaches as these students may not learn alternative approaches. Treatment with high-technology

Question for reflection

Patients at Sydney Children's Hospital now have access to magnetic resonance imaging (MRI) Medicare-eligible services at no cost through $5 million in funding from the Commonwealth government. The hospital has acquired an MRI machine and this service is now receiving Medicare funding. The government recognises the essential role of MRI in paediatric medicine. Children are more sensitive to radiation than adults and, unlike some other scans such as computed tomography and X-rays, MRI doesn't use ionising radiation. MRI uses intense magnetic fields to generate images. It is especially effective on soft tissue and as an aid in diagnosing diseases such as cancer. The Sydney Children's Hospital is a specialist facility for children's health and a paediatric teaching centre. It provides a comprehensive range of services for children throughout New South Wales. This is the fifth children's hospital to be granted Medicare eligibility following the Royal Children's Hospital (Brisbane), the Women's and Children's Hospital (Adelaide), the Princess Margaret Hospital for Children (Perth) and the Mater Children's Hospital (Brisbane). (Australian Government Department of Health and Ageing, 2006a)

How does this example of resource allocation reflect society's values and beliefs about the use of technology, children's lives and the role of prevention?

medicine is costly and these interventions may not result in a higher quality of life or improved health outcomes.

When considering the costs of health care provision, attention is drawn to the cost of investigative procedures—that is, procedures used to diagnose rather than prevent or treat illnesses. As discussed in Chapter 3, consumers increasingly have

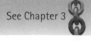

See Chapter 3

access to a broad range of information about health. However, health remains an expert domain and the idea of 'information asymmetry' points to the fact that the consumers of health care generally know less than those who provide it (Ross et al., 2005). One effect of this information asymmetry is that consumers are less able to differentiate between the quality of the services provided. Another effect of information asymmetry is that consumers need to trust the suppliers (in this case, health care providers), which may leave them vulnerable to supplier-induced demand. This increases the potential for moral hazard—the risk that the patient may receive more services than may be necessary. Examples where the risk of moral hazard increases include when health services are being paid for by a third party (government or insurance) or when doctors practise 'defensive medicine', whereby they cover all bases. Governments play a role by offering incentives that promote some choices over others—for example, subsidy of particular medications through the Pharmaceutical Benefits Scheme, or requiring consumers to provide a co-contribution to the cost of services. Information asymmetry and moral hazard drive the demand for curative health services and skew the expenditure away from preventative.

Health care: a collective or individual responsibility?

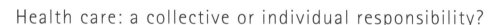

In Australia, the costs of health care are met through a mix of user-pays (whereby people using the health system pay some or all of the cost), public funding and private health insurance. Underlying these funding arrangements are debates about who should be responsible for paying for health care—individuals or the broader society. These debates are a reflection of social values that range from the individualistic to the collective. These values are evident in the philosophy of the two major political parties in Australia. The Australian Labor Party originated in the trade union movement and emphasises the role of government in achieving social justice, which extends to universal social rights to employment, education, health care and housing. Hence, health care policies that seek to strengthen the role of government in the provision of universal health care are generally proposed by the Labor Party because of its belief in collective responsibility. The Australian Liberal Party emphasises individual rights and freedoms, and the need for a lean government with minimal interference in the everyday lives of people. Further to this, it places emphasis on free enterprise and believes that the government should not compete with the private sector—hence the sale of government assets such as Telstra and the proposal to sell Medibank Private.

Historically, there have been major changes in policy direction in health care that can be understood as the result of a clash of ideologies of the two political parties, with the Labor Party favouring a universal (coverage for everyone) type of coverage and the Liberal Party following selective coverage (coverage for only those groups that are unable to provide for themselves). For example, in the 1970s, there were growing concerns about the rising costs of the infrastructure and resources required to support the predominantly biomedical model, and about the ability of this model to achieve equitable health care for all. The Whitlam Labor Federal Government's response to these concerns was to introduce the Community Health Program in 1973 and a universal health insurance program, Medibank, in 1975 (Milio, 1983). Despite a proliferation of services and programs, the Community Health Program did not achieve the aim of reforming the health care system and community health remained marginal to the hospital-focused health system (Butler, 2002). The Community Health Program disappeared with a change to the Fraser Coalition (Liberal and National Country Parties) Government in 1975 and was absorbed into general tax-sharing grants to the states. Medibank was not received favourably by doctors, private hospitals and private health insurers, and was gradually dismantled by the Fraser Government and re-established as a (government-owned) private insurance scheme in 1981 (Milio, 1983).

In the early 1980s, the tenets of primary health care were reintroduced into the broader Australian health policy debate by the newly elected Federal Labor Government, and in 1984 universal health insurance was reinstated as Medicare. The aim of the national health care funding system is to give universal access to health care through Medicare while also allowing for consumer choice from private-sector providers. Medicare is financed mostly from general taxation revenue, which includes a levy according to a person's taxable income, thus assuming a collective responsibility for health care. The level has been increased several times since 1984 and is currently set at 1.5 per cent of taxable income. The current Liberal Federal Government seeks to strengthen the role of private-sector involvement in health services provision and financing. This is evidenced by the 30 per cent subsidy introduced by the Federal Government for individuals to acquire private health insurance and other incentives to encourage their lifelong participation in private health insurance (e.g. higher premiums for people who join after the age of 30), and an increase in the Medicare levy for individuals on high incomes who do not have private health insurance. The current Federal Government argues that private-sector involvement promotes choice and individual responsibility for health costs (Financing and Analysis Branch, 2000).

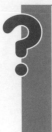

Questions for reflection

Should individuals be responsible for their own health insurance arrangements, or should universal health insurance cover the costs of health care provision? What are the issues that need to be taken into account in this debate?

Health expenditure

The reasons that governments become involved in the health system include the desire to address market failure (such as the provision of authoritative health information and public health services, e.g. immunisation) and broader social and political objectives (such as ensuring the provision of cost-effective and high-quality health services) (Ross et al., 2005). Some aspects of health are public goods, whereby the provision of these goods and services to the wider population benefits everyone—for example, provision of public hospitals and access to general practitioners at little or no cost. Governments also play a role in public health in an effort to minimise the factors that are detrimental to health and to promote healthy behaviours and a healthy environment.

In Australia, health expenditure represents approximately 9.7 per cent of GDP (in 2003–04) and it is estimated to rise to 16 per cent by 2044–45 because of the demand and supply pressures affecting health care (Productivity Commission, 2005). In 2003–04, total health expenditure was $78.6 billion, of which 68 per cent was funded by governments. Hospital services accounted for 34.8 per cent of recurrent health expenditure and public health (health promotion and disease prevention) accounted for 1.7 per cent. The areas experiencing rapid growth in terms of expenditure in the period 1997–98 to 2003–04 were aids and appliances (13.9 per cent per year on average), health research (12.5 per cent) and pharmaceuticals (11.7 per cent) (Australian Institute of Health and Welfare, 2006).

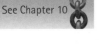

See Chapter 10

The Pharmaceutical Benefits Scheme (PBS) subsidises the costs of about 600 prescription medications listed in the pharmaceutical benefits schedule. Additional medications are added when assessed as meeting safety, quality, effectiveness and cost-effectiveness criteria. The process of gaining legitimacy for medications to be included in the schedule is a highly contested political activity. Government measures to slow down the growth of PBS costs are generally directed towards health consumers rather than health professionals. They include the introduction of a charge for health care cardholders in 1991, and charging additional amounts for premium brands when cheaper generic equivalents are available.

The allocation of health resources highlights the politics of health. Many of the policy debates in health relate to the allocation and control of scarce resources, rather than to efficacy of care. The priorities in health funding lead to the conclusion that we are funding an illness care system, rather than a health care system.

Questions for reflection

The Commonwealth Government listed Herceptin® (trastuzumab) on the Pharmaceutical Benefits Scheme (PBS) from 1 October 2006 for the treatment of patients with HER2 positive early stage breast cancer following surgery. Breast cancer is the most common cancer in women and affects 14,000 people per year. Of those, approximately 2000 people have HER2 positive breast cancer. In Australia, more than 2500 women died from the disease in 2001. Risk factors include age, alcohol consumption, certain chemicals, obesity and certain factors in a woman's fertility history. Herceptin® targets a particular type of breast cancer which produces an increased amount of a protein molecule called human epidermal growth factor receptor 2 (HER2). The HFR2 protein is associated with more aggressive disease and a poorer prognosis.

Treatment for early stage breast cancer normally consists of initial surgery, with or without radiotherapy, followed by chemotherapy drugs in combination. The addition of Herceptin® to existing treatment regimens will improve current treatment with a significant improvement in freedom from cancer recurrence. It is estimated that approximately 2000 people will commence Herceptin® in the first full financial year of listing for the treatment of early breast cancer. The listing of Herceptin® will add approximately $470 million to PBS and Repatriation Pharmaceutical Benefits Scheme expenditure between 2006–07 and 2009-10. (Australian Government Department of Health and Ageing, 2006b)

What are the vested interests of each of the key players (government, pharmaceutical companies, patients, treating physicians) in the listing of this medication?

How do these interests reflect the ideas about individual and collective responsibility for health care?

Who works in health: the health workforce

There is a great deal of interest in the size, distribution, composition and effectiveness of the Australian health workforce (Australian Institute of Health and Welfare, 2006). In 2005, the occupations with the greatest numbers were nurses (305,400) who comprised 54 per cent of the health workforce; medical practitioners (59,900) comprising 12 per cent of the workforce; dental workers (31,700), pharmacists (14,900), physiotherapists (14,300) and psychologists (13,900) (Australian Institute of Health and Welfare, 2006). Allied health professionals (physiotherapists, occupational therapists and podiatrists etc) (9 per cent) are the third-largest occupational grouping (Productivity Commission, 2005).

The news media often reports on the shortages of doctors and nurses, in particular, and the impact of these shortages on access to health care. The Australian Institute of Health and Welfare (2006) reports that the health workforce has been growing and experienced a 26 per cent increase from 2000 to 2005 (from 452,000 to 570,000 people). This growth rate far exceeds the population growth. The occupation involved in direct patient care that experienced the largest growth (89.5 per cent) was personal care and nursing assistants which increased in number from 36,100 to 68,500. However, some occupations did not share in this growth. For example, general practitioners, pharmacists and some allied health workers all experienced negative growth. Table 11.2 shows the factors that are impacting on health workforce trends.

Taking a sociological perspective to the health workforce raises two key questions: first, how are tasks allocated to the different health occupations; and second, why do some health occupations have greater legitimacy and status than others? In other words, how does the 'division of labour' and 'knowledge of professions' help to explain the social processes involved? Wearing (2004: 265) describes the division of labour as 'the way in which knowledge, skills, accomplishments and tasks are divided among the health occupations in the health care system as a whole'. Willis (1994) distinguishes between the technical division of labour that occurs within the health setting in relation to occupation and the social division of labour, which is a reflection of the wider social structure. Such a distinction enables exploration of the extent to which the division of labour is divided on the basis of technical skill or social status.

Classical theories about the division of labour refer to gender as a key determinant, suggesting that women's work in health care is an extension of their work within the home and is characterised by nurturing and caring. These accounts reflect a functionalist perspective that identifies gender attributes to explain the status and legitimacy of professions. Gender seems like an obvious basis for the division of health labour as females account for the bulk of the workforce in all health occupations, with the exception of medicine and dentistry

TABLE 11.2   Key developments and trends in the health workforce identified by the Productivity Commission (2005)

Workforce shortages	■ The Australian Medical Workforce Advisory Committee found an estimated shortage of between 800 to 1300 GPs in 2002
	■ The Australian Health Workforce Advisory Committee reported a shortfall of nurses requiring 10,000 to 12,000 new graduates in 2006
	■ The Department of Employment and Workplace Relations identified shortages across a range of health occupations
	■ Shortages are more pronounced in rural, remote and Indigenous communities
An older workforce	■ Between 1996 and 2001, the proportion of the health workforce aged over 45 years increased from 31 per cent to 39 per cent
	■ The proportion of the workforce aged over 45 years is 41 per cent of nurses, 46 per cent of the medical workforce, 43 per cent of dentists, 31 per cent of allied health and 27 per cent of medical imaging
Female-dominated	■ Apart from medicine and dentistry, females account for the bulk of the workforce in all health occupations
	■ Male-dominated professions of medicine and dentistry are becoming increasingly feminised
Some working fewer hours	■ More reliant on part-time workers than the wider workforce
	■ The most notable reduction in working hours has occurred within the medical profession
Increasing specialisation	■ Particularly in medicine and nursing
	■ This is significant because of the correlation between geographic location and specialisation—specialists tend to be located in major urban centres
Changing roles and scope of practice	■ Chronic diseases require a multidisciplinary approach to care
	■ Widening of scope of practice in areas of workforce shortages such as rural and remote

Source: Productivity Commission (2005); copyright of Commonwealth of Australia, reproduced with permission

(Productivity Commission, 2005). Viewed in this way, the lower status, lower rewards and subordinated nature of predominantly female-dominated health occupations such as nursing can be understood as the result of the dominance of the predominantly male medical profession in a patriarchal society.

Other theories about the division of labour focus on the way this is structured around a hierarchy of specialisation and differentiation. Willis (1994: 14) refers to the process of 'pass the task', whereby some occupations pass off mundane, routine or less challenging aspects of their work to 'lower-order' occupations. This viewpoint contributes to our understanding of the historical development of occupational territory—that is, how tasks that were once the exclusive domain of medicine become an accepted part of another health care worker's occupational territory. Sometimes this is unavoidable in certain work situations—for example, in the case of emergency situations or workforce shortages. However, as Willis (1994) points out, this process is not always consensual and is often the site of conflict and struggle as occupations seek to defend and extend their task domains. Thus, the medical profession is able to direct other health care workers through the hierarchical division of labour. The following section explores how the medical profession has achieved this level of dominance through its legitimation as a profession and strategies for maintaining its dominance.

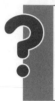

Question for reflection

Are tasks allocated to different health care occupations based on education and training or other factors?

Professions and professionalisation

Taken-for-granted understandings of what is meant by a profession usually include reference to educational standards, rigorous training, high level of skill and professional ethics or discipline. However, a closer examination of the work practices of different occupational groups suggests that what primarily distinguishes professions from other occupations is the extent to which they have been able to achieve government-regulated and sanctioned autonomy over their work—that is, freedom from having their work practices directed or controlled by those outside the profession. Professionals have a high degree of individual autonomy and protection from outside evaluation of their occupational territory. This is achieved through governments continuing to endorse an occupation as a profession.

Classical studies of professions have been preoccupied with identifying the characteristics that define an occupation as a profession. This is known as the trait approach and a range of traits have been identified (see, for example, Table 11.3). The most common traits identified for health professionals include a scientific body of knowledge, high standard of education and accreditation of its members. From the perspective of the 'trait approach', occupations seeking legitimacy as professions must adopt professionalisation strategies, such as developing a knowledge base, tertiary education and gaining occupational control of their work. However, the trait approach cannot account for the failure of some occupations to be recognised as professions, even when they meet these 'professional criteria'. Evetts (2006) argues that more recently there has been a move from *defining* a profession towards the *concept* of professionalism. She argues that this more fruitfully allows exploration of 'how and in what ways the discourse of professionalism is being used (by states, by employers and managers, and by some relatively powerful occupational groups themselves) as an instrument of occupational change (including resistance to change and social control)' (Evetts, 2006: 141).

TABLE 11.3   Characteristics of a profession

The occupation is based on a systematic body of theoretical knowledge	This means that not only is there a set of highly specialised skills, but also a cohesive body of abstract, organised, scientific knowledge.
The occupation is authoritative in its area of expertise	The judgments of persons, especially clients, are subordinate to those of the professional.
The occupation has a monopoly of practice in its area of expertise	This monopoly is formally sanctioned by society, usually in the form of a legal charter. Under these conditions, only the profession itself can say who will and who will not practice. The community agrees to control those who attempt to practice who are not members. In addition, the profession controls or polices its own members.
The occupation maintains ethical conduct	The members of the occupation adhere to a code of ethics that regulates their behaviour.

Adapted with permission from *Sociology One*, Waters Crook © Pearson Education Australia (1993).

Thus, taking a 'concept of professionalism' approach requires consideration of two related dimensions: a task-related component and the resultant social practices. With regard to medicine, both these dimensions can be applied to understanding its professional status. The medical profession has ownership of a body of knowledge and skills that demarcates its occupational territory, defining its tasks and practices. The state further legitimises the role of the medical profession by authorising the 'official' role of doctors in social practices such as the issuing of sick leave certificates, death certificates, workers compensation, etc.

The ideas, values and beliefs that surround professionalism have been influential in legitimising the position of the medical profession at the top of the hierarchical division of health labour. Willis (1994) links the ideology of professionalism with the ideology of expertise, suggesting that doctors have expert knowledge and therefore this supports their claim to legitimacy and their right (authority) to control the division of health labour. Education and training play a pivotal role in the professionalisation of medicine because they ensure that knowledge and skills are passed on to others; they expand the extent of knowledge and skills through technical developments and research; and they are an important part of the socialisation of new doctors into the medical profession (Wearing, 2004).

Question for reflection

What factors do you believe are most important in defining an occupation as a profession?

Medical dominance

Our health system is well suited to the dominance of one profession that is the legitimated expert on health. Within our health system there is sufficient, even over, demand for health services, which ensures that the provision of private health care by doctors will continue to be supported by market forces. The market for cures is highly competitive; however, the medical profession has a competitive advantage as its legitimacy is based on scientific proof. Members of the medical profession are also able to build upon notions of trust in expert knowledge, particularly when health and illness are individualised. In our society, the medical profession is also fortunate to have state patronage, which has ensured that its members have become institutionalised experts on all matters related to health.

A key feature of the health system in our society is medical dominance, which refers to 'the social and historical dominance of the division of health labour and the health system by the medical profession including medical knowledge and research' (Wearing, 2004: 262; see also Willis, 1989). This dominance is exerted through the medical profession's ability to organise and control the provision of health services. Willis (1994) describes how the division of health labour is sustained at three levels: autonomy (doctors direct and control their own work); authority (doctors are authorised to direct the work of others); and medical sovereignty (doctors are considered the health experts in wider society). We can see many examples of this in society today. For example, in the welfare sector, the evidence that doctors provide on issues relating to the ability of a person to retrain or the types of work that a person might do is important in assessing the person's entitlement to a disability support pension. In the area of occupational health, doctors play a significant role in writing medical certificates to legitimate work absences or by diagnosing compensable injuries or diseases.

Willis (1994) explains that the positions of various occupations within the hierarchy are the result of medical dominance that is exerted in four different ways. First, medicine remains dominant through directing the work of other health care providers in the health care system, known as subordination. There are several examples of how medicine has controlled other health care providers. For example, midwifery was predominantly a female-dominated profession, which was taken over and subordinated by the medical profession. Midwives can now only practice under the control of a medical practitioner.

The second way that medicine maintains its dominance is by limiting the amount of autonomy an allied health professional can have. Limitation involves restriction of the occupational territory in which the occupation can intervene. Examples of limitation include optometry and pharmacy. This restriction may be to a particular part of the body (as with optometry) or to utilising a specific therapeutic technique (as with pharmacy). Registration acts specify exactly what constitutes the occupational territory of these occupations, including techniques and diagnostic aids that may be used, while at the same time exempting medical practitioners from the provisions of the acts. The acts themselves have been the result of lengthy negotiations and struggles in which medical lobbying has played a prominent part. For example, optometrists can provide us with glasses, but cannot prescribe medication if we have conjunctivitis. Radiographers cannot legally interpret the X-rays they take.

Medicine also exercises its dominance through resistance to occupations seeking to enter the 'legitimate' health sector. This process is known as exclusion and it is most obvious in the case of alternative therapies. For example, naturopathy has been resisted by the medical profession and in effect is regarded as a 'deviant medical occupation' because it does not have the same legitimacy as orthodox medicine (Gort & Coburn, 1988).

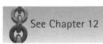 See Chapter 12

The fourth way that medicine exercises its domination of health care professions is through the process of incorporation. In this process, medicine expands its occupational territory or scope of practice to take over the work of others. For example, Eastwood (2000) found that general practitioners (GPs) in Australia are increasingly incorporating complementary and alternative medicine (CAM)—particularly acupuncture, manipulation, hypnosis, vitamin therapy, herbal treatments and homeopathy—into mainstream primary care. The motive for GPs to incorporate CAM into their practice is not just in response to consumer demand. Eastwood (2000) demonstrated that it is also linked to economic globalisation (through consumerist ideology and cultural commodification), consumer demand for choice and GPs themselves being disenchanted with modernist medical science.

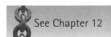 See Chapter 12

Question for reflection

Which do you think is most influential in maintaining medical dominance—subordination, limitation, exclusion or incorporation?

Threats to medical dominance

Even though there is strong evidence of the existence of medical dominance, medicine does not completely dominate health care. The following discussion outlines the ways that medical dominance is constrained, resisted and challenged by other players in the health care system.

The Australian constitution prevents any form of civil conscription of medicine, which provides the medical profession with a high level of autonomy or control over its profession. However, the government still plays a role in legitimating health care and in this way it has some influence over the medical profession, usually as an attempt to restrain or reduce costs. For example, the Federal Government closely monitors Medicare expenditure through its National Compliance Program and Professional Services Review scheme and by encouraging people to report fraud. The object of these strategies is to protect the community from the risks associated with inappropriate practice and to protect the Commonwealth from higher costs. These types of legislation and associated strategies serve to monitor the practice of the medical profession closely and they result in serious consequences for those who breach these laws. These processes could be viewed as deprofessionalisation strategies, as they undermine the credibility of the medical profession in the eyes of the public, resulting in scepticism and diminished trust (Germov, 2005). They represent a threat to the political autonomy and self-regulation of the medical profession.

There is evidence that governments exercise bureaucratic control over the work of medical practitioners. These developments can be explained through theories of proletarianisation or corporatisation, which refer to processes whereby corporate managers and bureaucratic regulations reduce the amount of control that doctors have over their work (Germov, 2005). In recent years, the Federal Government has increasingly sought to influence and shape the form of medical practice, and general practice in particular. For example, the Federal Government introduced the Practice Incentives Program in 1998 to encourage the uptake of initiatives that improve the quality of care, such as computerisation, after hours care, teaching and participation in the quality use of medicines program. Other initiatives, such as the introduction of new item numbers for care planning and case management, seek to improve patient care for older patients and those with chronic or complex health issues (Australian Government Department of Health and Ageing, 2007b). These incentives and allowances influence the way that GPs work. For example, they encourage GPs to work more collaboratively with other service providers and to consider patient care as a continuous rather than episodic process.

The media also has a role to play in the deprofessionalisation of medicine. In stark contrast to the breaches of the *Health Insurance Act 1973*, which mostly pass unnoticed by the general public, is the widespread media exposure of medical negligence. A recent example was the 'Doctor Death' headlines associated with Dr Jayant Patel, who allegedly made a number of serious errors ranging from performing the wrong procedure to causing death while working as a surgeon at Bundaberg Base Hospital in Queensland. In addition to the high-profile episodes of medical negligence, there are many thousands of instances of adverse events, which are mostly preventable, that do not result in litigation. These cases cause concern among the general public and result in a lack of confidence about the skills and abilities of the medical profession.

Medical dominance is also challenged by increasing divisions and specialisations within medicine. The traditional divide between medicine and surgery has become even more fragmented within these broad categories. For example, within medicine there are cardiologists, endocrinologists, gastro-enterologists, geriatricians and general physicians. There are also specialties that arise in response to disease types—for example, oncologists for cancer care. Within the field of surgery, there are specialty areas such as orthopaedics, cardiothoracic, urology, oro-facial and vascular surgeons. The fragmentation that has occurred through specialisation serves to diversify the interests within the medical profession. As a result, the medical profession is not one interest group, but many, which may potentially weaken the power of the profession. In addition, rather than speaking as one voice on health care, alternative views have been established. For example, the Doctors Reform Society, which has different views to the Australian Medical Association (AMA), was established because groups of doctors were disenchanted with the activities of the AMA.

As well as the role of the medical practitioner being carved into various specialties, there is also a move from new professionals and para-professionals to take over the domain of medicine. This is being driven by other health occupations that want to extend their occupational territory, as well as by governments that are seeking to meet the increasing demand for health care with a limited workforce supply. The measures they employ may include the development of new professions. For example, there has been considerable debate about the development of the nurse practitioner role, particularly in light of evidence that nurses can effectively deliver routine management of chronic conditions (Laurant et al., 2004). In the USA and the United Kingdom, there have been moves to introduce the role of physician assistants or medical care practitioners (respectively) who are health care professionals licensed to practice medicine under physician supervision (Parle et al., 2006).

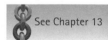 See Chapter 13

CONCLUSION

The health system and the professions that work within it are under increasing pressure to meet demands for health care with a limited supply of resources and workforce. The overriding concern of governments will be to contain expenditure, with the current estimate that health expenditure could rise to as much as 16 per cent of GDP by 2044–45. National policy initiatives such as Medicare will come under increasing scrutiny, particularly when we consider that Medicare was established when hospitals and doctors dominated the health system. The expansion of community-based care and the increasing size of the non-medical workforce will test the ability of this system to provide universal access to health care.

With rising incomes, people will spend more and expect more from health services. Demographic changes such as an increasing proportion of people aged over 65 years will significantly impact on health service provision and expenditure. For example, spending on those aged over 65 years is currently around four times more per person than on those aged less than 65. The incidence of chronic disease is increasing with ageing—for example, type two diabetes and dementia—which will be a major contributor to changing care needs. New models of health care that focus on prevention, social determinants and community care are part of the response to these factors. However, these responses also challenge the dominance of the acute care (hospital) system and the central place of the medical practitioner.

The average age of health workers is increasing and service providers will be seeking to replace greater numbers of retiring workers and secure additional labour to meet accelerating demand in an environment where growth in effective labour supply is expected to be slower than population growth. There is likely to be considerable expansion of the role of allied health personnel, alternative health practitioners and the development of new roles as consumers exert their influence within the health system and the current trends in expanding occupational territory and substitution of medical care continue. Technological change will continue to be an important contributor to growing demand for and spending on health care—different models of care and new workforce practices will be required to accommodate and utilise the wider range of treatment possibilities.

REVIEW QUESTIONS

1. Are debates about health more about allocation of scarce resources than about efficacy of care?
2. How should governments address the issue raised by workforce shortages in health?
3. To what extent is medical dominance threatened in a contemporary health care system?

KEY TERMS

Autonomy, authority, medical sovereignty
Deprofessionalisation
Information asymmetry
Legitimacy
Medical dominance
Moral hazard

Occupational territory
Professions, professionalisation
Proletarianisation/corporatisation
Subordination, limitation, exclusion,
    incorporation
Trait approach

FURTHER READING

Australian Institute of Health and Welfare 2006, *Australia's Health 2006*, Canberra, Australian Institute of Health and Welfare.

Belcher, H. 2005, 'Power, politics and health care', in Germov, J. (ed.), *Second Opinion: An Introduction to Health Sociology*, South Melbourne, Oxford University Press, pp. 267–89.

George, J. and Davis, A. 1998, *States of Health: Health and Illness in Australia*, South Melbourne, Longman.

Germov, J. 2005, 'Challenges to medical dominance', in Germov, J. (ed.), *Second Opinion: Introduction to Health Sociology*, South Melbourne, Oxford University Press, pp. 290–313.

Wearing, M. 2004, 'Medical dominance and the division of labour in the health professions', in Grbich, C. (ed.), *Health in Australia: Sociological Concepts and Issues*, Frenchs Forest, Pearson Education Australia.

Willis, E. 1989, *Medical Dominance*, St. Leonards, Allen & Unwin.

Willis, E. 1994, *Illness and Social Relations: Issues in the Sociology of Health Care*, St Leonards, Allen & Unwin.

Chapter 12

Complementary and Alternative Medicine

Introduction

In February 2004, the then Premier of Tasmania, Jim Bacon, publicly announced that he had lung cancer. He had been a heavy smoker and hoped that by making his diagnosis public, he would contribute to the anti-smoking campaign. After this announcement, Mr Bacon received 157 pieces of correspondence that suggested the use of complementary and alternative medicine (CAM); however, he had no interest in this type of treatment. These pieces of correspondence were analysed by the Director of Medical Oncology at the Royal Hobart Hospital, Professor Lowenthal, and published in the Medical Journal of Australia. Lowenthal (2005: 578) found that 'many of these unsolicited communications recommended a variety of unorthodox treatment.' Some of the treatments were found to either be harmful (Laetrile, Hoxsey, coffee enemas) or of no benefit (shark cartilage, glyconutrients), and others had some evidence of benefit (meditation, reishi mushrooms, mangosteen plants). Lowenthal (2005) found fourteen pieces of correspondence that asked Mr Bacon to contact the correspondent for further information about 'secret methods' and some of these requested a fee for information. Lowenthal argued that this points to the potential dangers of CAM treatments and the need for physicians to be aware that their patients may be receiving advice about these treatments, which is indicative of the need for 'authoritative evidence-based information' (2005: 576).

Health care systems are shaped by the larger political, economic and socio-cultural settings within which they are embedded. This chapter focuses on how the availability of alternative or complementary methods of health care contributes to the development of our health care system. The provision of alternative health care has been strongly resisted by the orthodox medical system. However, with the increasing use of alternative and complementary modalities (some of which are practised by medical practitioners), there is a range of issues to consider. A sociological approach to CAM explores how the use and acceptance of these healing modalities change over time; how they interact with orthodox medicine; and, in particular, the processes of power, legitimacy, inclusion and exclusion that serve to differentiate complementary and alternative medicine from orthodox medicine.

Objectives

After reading this chapter, you should be able to:

■ explain the reasons for the changing relationship between complementary and alternative medicines and orthodox medicine
■ understand politico-legal and clinical legitimacy and how these processes influence the acceptance and use of complementary and alternative medicines
■ critically analyse the reasons why complementary and alternative medicine have increased in popularity.

What are complementary and alternative medicines?

It is difficult to categorically define complementary and alternative medicines, commonly referred to by the acronym CAM. The broad range of health care services and products includes self-care according to folk principles, care rendered in an organised health care system based on alternative traditions or practices, and products purchased over-the-counter or prescribed by practitioners. Connor (2004: 1697) defines complementary and alternative medicine as 'those healing modalities that are not part of state-authorised biomedical services, but which are offered on a fee-for-service basis by other practitioners with varying types of training and certification, such as chiropractors, naturopaths, masseurs, iridologists, and acupuncturists'. Some of these services and products are well known and others are viewed as more obscure or exotic (e.g. Filipino psychic surgery, visual imaging). Clavarino and Yates (1995: 253) explain:

> They have derived from a wide variety of sources, including ethnic and folk traditions (e.g., herbalism); established religions or semi-religious cults (e.g., faith healing in its varied forms); philosophies (e.g., traditional Chinese medicine); metaphysical movements (e.g., crystal healing); or as a response to, or in connection with mainstream medical practice (e.g., homeopathy, osteopathy, chiropractic).

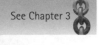
See Chapter 3

The Therapeutic Goods Administration in Australia classifies complementary medicines as herbal, homeopathic, traditional (Chinese, Ayurvedic), vitamins and minerals, nutritional supplements and aromatherapy products.

Alternative therapies draw on quite different concepts of health to orthodox medicine. Disease is central to orthodox medicine—for example, health is defined as the absence of disease. Disease is usually conceived as being within the individual body or body part. Diagnosis is focused around the structure and form of organisms that indicate a deviation from normal functioning. Therapy aims to destroy or suppress disease. By contrast, alternative therapies focus on health as a balance, a definition of disease is focused around bodily attempts to rid it of toxic substances, diagnosis focuses on 'reading the body' and therapy is aimed at strengthening the vitalising, positive forces within the body (Barry & Yuill, 2002: 49).

The stark differences between the healing practices of CAM and orthodox Western medicine have led studies to focus on the two as dichotomous—that is, in terms of either/or. In defining these healing modalities, language plays an important role in giving meaning, particularly regarding the relationship of CAM with orthodox medicine. In recent years, writers in the area and health care practitioners prefer to use the term complementary to alternative. Alternative implies a choice between two modalities. Complementary suggests that the two modalities work within the same system, where one practice is complementary to, rather than alternative from, the other. However, some research has demonstrated that consumers of CAM do not view the two models in this way (for example, Connor, 2004: 1698). Rather, CAM could be viewed as 'additional' (Murray & Shepherd, 1993), or Connor (2004) refers to it as 'mixed therapy regimes'. Other terms that are gaining in popularity are 'integrated' (in the United Kingdom) and 'integrative' (in the USA). Further, research by Lew-Ting (2005) found that some approaches to health-seeking practices result in a blend of biomedicine and CAM, which he refers to as 'hybrid medicine'. These terms are used in a relational sense and the inference is that these therapies sit outside of orthodox medicine, but more often in a way that supplements or augments rather than replaces it.

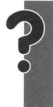

Question for reflection

What term do you think best encapsulates the relationship between CAM and orthodox medicine—complementary, alternative, additional, mixed therapy regime, integrative, integrated, hybrid or other?

Legitimacy

As can be seen from the above section, complementary and alternative medicines have become increasingly intermingled with the biomedical model in Western societies. Turner (2004) questions whether the growth in the acceptance of CAM is the result of mainstreaming, co-opting or neutralising. Central to these theories for the increasing use of CAM is the notion of legitimacy. Legitimation is defined as a process 'whereby a set of practices is accepted as authoritative and becomes dominant through the political process of justification' (Willis, 1994: 55). A distinction is made between politico-legal legitimacy, where there is official recognition by the state; scientific legitimacy, whereby there is evidence to prove efficacy; and clinical legitimacy, which refers to acceptance and use by the public.

The quest for politico-legal legitimacy is hard-fought as the rewards are great, particularly in a health market where the demand for services is ever increasing. Connor's (2004: 1697) definition of CAM above draws our attention to the way that CAMs are generally excluded from the state-funded health care system by describing them as 'not part of state-authorised biomedical services'. State support for CAM would entail the provision of Medicare benefits and provider numbers to other health professionals. The Cochrane Collaboration makes explicit the political and socio-cultural processes involved in excluding CAM from the mainstream by describing CAM as 'a broad domain of healing resources that encompasses all health systems, modalities and practices and their accompanying theories and beliefs, other than those intrinsic to the politically dominant health system of a particular society or culture in a given historical period' (Panel on Definition and Description CRMCA1, 1997). Legitimising CAM as a part of conventional medicine is a highly political process and one that is strongly resisted by the medical profession.

See Chapter 2

See Chapter 11

By looking through a sociological lens, we become aware of the process of medicalisation whereby the biomedical approach reaches further into our lives. In addition, due to the dominance of medicine that exists within our health care system, the medical profession is viewed as the most authoritative source of information about health. These two factors combine to create resistance to, and less opportunity for, CAM. Doctors enjoy socially legitimated high status and while this may not be enough to stop people from using CAM, it can make it more difficult for people to seek alternatives to the biomedical model. Although alternative practitioners have some political-legal legitimacy, this is tenuous when compared to their biomedical counterparts. Baer (2006: 1781) claims that 'While complementary practitioners, including naturopaths but particularly chiropractors and osteopaths, have indeed improved their legitimacy within the context of the Australian dominative medical system, this development has not seriously eroded biomedical domination '.

Thus, the extent to which a CAM modality sits alongside or outside the dominant model of health may influence its likelihood of achieving legitimacy. For example, Baer (2006) argues that chiropractors and osteopaths have taken on a certain orthodoxy. They maintain membership of their own professional associations but tend not to belong to other complementary medicine associations (Baer, 2006). Meeker and Haldeman (2002) argue that much of the success of chiropractic's quest for legitimacy has been the result of research efforts and improvement of its educational and licensing systems. Thus, through prolonged investigation of spinal manipulation, chiropractic has begun to establish scientific legitimacy. Using this example, Baer (2006) argues that the quest for legitimacy can be adversely affected when a therapy is subsumed under the bigger umbrella of natural therapies, or even complementary therapies. Thus, association with all other modalities included in the broad label of CAM serves to distance it from the orthodoxy, thus limiting the chances of legitimacy.

An essential requirement for gaining acceptance within the realm of biomedicine is the provision of scientific forms of evidence—scientific legitimacy. Barry (2006: 2647) describes evidence in this context as 'therapeutic efficacy for biomedically diagnosed disorders, within the individual body (or body part), and as measurable utilising science-based research strategies, most notably the randomised control trial'. However, Barry's (2006) research demonstrates that the randomised control trial is antithetical to CAM and not capable of generating evidence of efficacy, apart from the physical experience. For example, people with the same biomedical condition (e.g. rhinitis) may receive different homeopathic remedies according to their total symptom picture, thus the application of a double blind randomised control trial to assess the efficacy of homeopathy for the treatment of rhinitis is contrary to the prescription of individualised remedies (Barry, 2006).

Orthodox medicine claims that the rising use of CAM raises the critical issue of safety (Myers & Cheras, 2004). This 'framing' of CAM as inherently unsafe and the privileging of scientific knowledge as the sole source of evidence tends to be made on the assumption that orthodox medicine is completely safe. Particular concerns are expressed about the potential for adverse reactions. The *Medical Journal of Australia* reported a case of accidental death from acute selenium poisoning that occurred after a 75-year-old man self-administered sodium selenite powder in an effort to prevent prostate cancer (See et al., 2006). The article aimed to illustrate the risks of failing to critically evaluate Internet information and to expose the myth that natural therapies are inherently safe. Doctors are also concerned about the unknown interaction of CAMs with conventional medicines. For example, patients are advised to stop taking herbal preparations up to six weeks pre-operatively. Research by MacLennan et al. (2006) found that almost half of their respondents took conventional medicines as well as CAMs on the day of their operation; however, 57.2 per cent did not report the use of CAMs to their doctor.

The framing of CAM as unsafe by orthodox medicine contrasts with the strength of dominant ideas that equate CAM with nature. The general belief is that these alternatives are natural and therefore safe, even though their safety has not been assured through the scientific process. About half of those involved in research by MacLennan et al. (2006) assumed (incorrectly) that CAMs were independently tested by a government agency. In Australia, most CAM products are listed (required to meet safety and quality of manufacturing guidelines) but not registered (evaluated for quality, safety and efficacy). Clearly, there is a substantial gap between consumer beliefs about CAM use and the strength of scientific evidence supporting its use (Bensoussan & Lewith, 2004). These safety concerns strengthen the call for evidence of efficacy, safety and quality of CAMs; however, the methodological difficulties inherent in the application of biomedical scientific testing to CAMs will require a multipronged approach that takes account of the multifaceted nature of CAM use.

The application and acceptance of experiential knowledge of CAM in the debate about efficacy is known as 'clinical legitimacy'. Members of the general public tend to be less concerned about scientific verification and more concerned with their own experience as evidence of efficacy. If the patient experiences improvement as a result of their use of CAM, then this serves to legitimise the treatment. Thus, in the debates about politico-legal and clinical legitimacy, the importance of clinical legitimacy cannot be underestimated as a motivating force for the continued use of CAM. The strength of clinical legitimacy also highlights the differences between lay legitimacy and professional/scientific legitimacy.

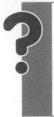

Questions for reflection

What factors are most likely to influence your decision to use CAM?
How do these fit with the different notions of legitimacy—politico-legal, scientific or clinical?

Professionalisation of complementary and alternative medicines

See Chapter 11

In drawing on the discussion in Chapter 11 about professions, this section explores the strategies towards professionalism engaged in by CAM practitioners. Strategies towards professionalism are strongly influenced by the dominant discourses of science, evidence and legitimacy. As pointed out in Chapter 11, the general characteristics of a profession are a scientific body of knowledge, high standard of education and accreditation of its members.

Many CAM practitioners hold university degrees or diplomas from specialist colleges; however, due to the diversity of the field, there is not an exclusive domain of knowledge that is relevant only to CAM, which limits the ability to claim a specific body of knowledge for CAM as a whole. This is not to deny that there is some knowledge that is very specific and specialised to particular CAM practices— for example, homeopathy. Another problem created by the diversity within CAM is the potential for overlapping boundaries around their knowledge claims. This leads to contestation over boundaries and who has the most credible knowledge claim (Welsh et al., 2004). Some CAM practices align themselves more closely with science to achieve these aims. For example, homeopathy and chiropractic have conducted scientific investigations in an attempt to achieve scientific legitimacy and therefore a claim to a specific body of knowledge (Cant, 1996). The demarcation of knowledge is an important step towards professionalisation but in a field as diverse as CAM, it can also serve to further divide and differentiate.

As well as the need for the development of a knowledge base for CAM and for the practices within CAM, professionalisation strategies also seek to differentiate

CAM knowledge from that of orthodox medicine. The medical profession has exerted its dominance through strategies that maintain its monopoly position, particularly in relation to its state-endorsed legitimacy. In response to this, CAM providers have sought to increase their status and share of the health care market. Hirschkorn (2006: 534) argues that 'knowledge claims, while not necessarily the determinants of professional status, represent a key vehicle through which these struggles are rhetorically played out, particularly with regard to science'. She explains that much of CAM knowledge is unrecognised by orthodox medicine as it is outside of its scientific paradigm and in order to become recognised, it needs to be more 'scientific' (Hirschkorn, 2006). However, this creates a paradox whereby on the one hand CAM distinguishes itself by its non-scientific nature and therein lies much of the consumer appeal, and on the other hand the professionalisers within CAM are seeking to increase their professional status by achieving scientific legitimacy, which may in turn affect its wider appeal. Conversely, the orthodox medical profession is moving towards embracing the holistic nature of CAM, but at the same time moving towards evidence-based medicine.

Even with high levels of education, CAM practitioners are not readily perceived as knowledgeable or credible experts on health, primarily because of medical dominance. The persistence of stigmatising labels such as 'quacks' is a significant barrier to obtaining credibility (Saks, 2003). CAM practitioners argue that a key strategy for professionalism is centred around educating the public about their role and level of expert knowledge, and gaining credibility within the mainstream health system. However, tension remains because this is linked to the need for scientific legitimacy and to ensure that therapies and practices are evidence-based (Kelner et al., 2004).

Moves towards regulation in Australia have encouraged membership of professional organisations and associations such as the Australian Traditional Medicine Society, although there are over 100 such organisations in Australia (Expert Committee on Complementary Medicines in the Health System, 2003). As evident from the earlier discussion in this chapter, there is great diversity among CAM practices and practitioners. These factors make it difficult for CAM practitioners to progress the professionalisation of their occupation collectively. Inherent in the regulation process is the need for standardisation—both in terms of education and practice. Baer (2006) explains that in the case of naturopathy, this may be difficult to achieve because of its eclectic nature and philosophical diffusiveness, which in turn means that the scope of practice changes over time. In addition to the difficulties in relation to developing cohesiveness within CAM, there is also resistance from the established health care professions to encouraging CAM groups towards self-regulation (Kelner et al., 2004).

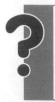

Question for reflection

Can CAM practitioners achieve professional status? Give reasons for your answer.

Who is likely to use complementary and alternative medicines?

The stereotypes and myths that exist about users of CAM suggest that they are people who seek alternative lifestyles ('hippies') or have rejected mainstream society, including orthodox medicine. However, research about the people who use CAM does not support these views. Estimates of the number of Australian people who use CAM vary, although recent reports place it at about half of the population. The results of the National Health Survey conducted in Australia every five years indicate that the number of people using CAM is increasing. For example, in 1995, only 1.3 per cent of people reported consulting a chiropractor in the two weeks prior to the survey, compared to 16 per cent in 2005 (Australian Bureau of Statistics, 2006). This most recent survey shows that a significant proportion of people who use medications for some chronic illnesses, reported using vitamin, minerals or herbal treatments (arthritis/osteoporosis 64 per cent, mental illness 57 per cent) (Australian Bureau of Statistics, 2006). It is claimed that a socio-behavioural model can help to increase our understanding of the interplay of belief, socio-demographic and individual factors on health care decisions. According to this model, the factors that determine health care seeking behaviour include a predisposition to use health services (beliefs, demographic and social variables); ability to secure health services (e.g. income); and medical need (Andersen and Newman, 1973 cited in Sirois and Gick, 2002).

While there are some similarities between users of CAM, it is important to acknowledge that they are not a homogenous group. For example, Sirois and Gick (2002) argue that those who use CAM long term may have different characteristics from those who use CAM initially but not over a sustained period of time. They claim these variations are lost in dichotomous comparisons with CAM users and non-CAM users. Similarly, Adams et al. (2003) found that while women are more likely to use CAM, they are not a homogenous group—for example, CAM use differed with age and geographic location. Research has identified particular socio-demographic characteristics and illness profiles that are associated with CAM use. People who use CAM are more likely to be female, younger than conventional users, have a higher level of education and have higher income (Adams et al., 2003; Easthope, 2005; Zollman & Vickers, 1999).

People who use CAM also tend to have poorer health status and higher rates of chronic conditions. They are seeking to use CAM for a greater number of physical symptoms, symptoms of greater intensity and longer disease duration (MacLennan et al., 2006; Robotin & Penman, 2006; Sirois & Gick, 2002).

Many reasons have been put forward for the growth in the use and acceptance of CAM, ranging from dissatisfaction with conventional medicine to philosophical beliefs and values about life that are congruent with CAM. Dissatisfaction with the health outcomes of orthodox medicine is one of the major reasons provided for the increasing popularity of CAM. Consumers become dissatisfied primarily because orthodox medicine does not always eradicate suffering and provide good health (Siahpush, 1998). For example, the problem of iatrogenesis (illnesses caused by medical intervention) is widely reported. Easthope (2005) claims that the illnesses of modern societies are more likely to be either chronic or terminal and, by definition, these disease states cannot be cured, which is the objective of the biomedical model. As a result, the limits of biomedicine are exposed, which reduces consumer confidence in the efficacy of conventional medicine. For example, the inability of biomedicine to cure many illnesses (e.g. cancer, AIDS) or to alleviate the symptoms of other illnesses satisfactorily (e.g. chronic pain conditions such as arthritis) may lead some people to seek alternatives.

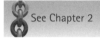
See Chapter 2

Another motivating factor for the use of CAM is dissatisfaction with elements of doctor–patient interaction. Some consumers claim that '[d]octors adopt a materialistic instead of service oriented ideology and opt for a doctor-centred pattern of relationship instead of one that is characterised by mutual participation' (Siahpush, 1998). Research indicates that people who use CAM are unwilling to accept the power differentials that exist between them and their health care provider, and less likely to be passive recipients of care (Siahpush, 1998). For some there is a perception of a more egalitarian relationship between consumers and CAM practitioners. McClean (2005) explains that the individualistic, depersonalised, biomedical and reductionist approach to health is conducive to blaming the individual for their own health. While CAM therapies may also locate the cause of disease within the individual, this is done to promote 'creativity, innovation and empowerment in the healing act and provides healers and patients with greater agency and control in the construction of healing reality, and does not just lead to "victim-blaming"' (McClean, 2005: 644).

Connor (2004: 1702) refers to healing as a moral relationship as well as a technical or social one. In this way, moral discourses of fraud, deception and immoral behaviour may permeate healing relationships. Media coverage of impropriety among members of the medical profession serves to tarnish their reputation and lead to distrust. Allsop (2006: 626) explains that '[d]issatisfaction with a doctor's competence or behaviour, although it is about particular doctors, may have a radiating effect on the profession as a whole'. Diminishing trust in the medical profession is a key feature of the deprofessionalisation theory, which predicts that the power of the medical profession declines as a result of this and the public's increased education and awareness of health issues (Germov, 2005). Thus, the decline in the status of medicine makes room for the possibility of seeking assistance from an alternative expert on health.

See Chapter 11

We also need to understand the increasing popularity of CAM as a reflection of the broader social and political processes of our society. We live in what is characterised as a postmodern society, where social life is different to that characterised by social structures of class, gender and culture, with new ideas about nature, science and technology, health, authority, individual responsibility and consumerism (Siahpush, 1998). We also live in a globalised society, where information from sources such as the Internet is not confined to specific powerful groups. Additionally there is a focus on consumption. We are identified by our consuming practices (e.g. fashion, wearing of brand names) rather than our social class position. In such a context, the types of health practices and the values that we place around different models of health are also likely to change. Philosophies such as self-determination, choice and individualism lead people to see health as a responsibility for individuals to take control, and to purchase consumer goods to attain health.

Recognising these social forces helps us to understand why CAM holds intuitive appeal for those with holistic beliefs and a preference for this approach to care. This preference can be understood as a rejection of the reductionist nature of biomedicine and its focus on health as the absence of disease. Goldner (2004) found that participants in her study emphasised the way CAM takes account of the 'whole' person, including mental, emotional and spiritual concerns and health as well-being. CAM practitioners offer a 'natural' alternative that is holistic and promotes active participation in the healing process.

Further, it is argued that part of the attraction of alternative medicine is its association with the natural world and the healing power of nature. This is partly due to the increased perception of risk in postmodern society that is caused by high technology responses to health. Connor (2004: 1699) refers to the symbolic value of natural therapies, explaining that 'being "natural" signifies a lack of danger or risk that renders these therapies more amenable to personal decision-making and control rather than professional medical surveillance'. Conversely, the symbolic value of pharmaceuticals is as toxic therapies (Connor, 2004: 1700). These viewpoints are informed by a 'green culture' (Bakx, 1991), within which the body is viewed as an extension of nature, and an 'antiscience' perspective (Kurz, 1994) whereby there is suspicion and distrust of science and technology.

A recurring theme in the research about CAM relates to the expectation that individuals will take responsibility for their health. For consumers to take more responsibility for their own health, they need to be empowered to do so.

This again emphasises the importance of the relationship between the consumer and the practitioner, and the more egalitarian nature of relationships between consumers and CAM practitioners compared with patients and doctors (Goldner, 2004). Individuals who want to take a proactive approach to their health make the shift from passive patient to active consumer. These people are more likely to find explanations of causes of ill health in the context of individual lifestyle and are therefore amenable to change. What must be considered here, however, is that CAM, like biomedicine, does not take account of the structural causes of ill health and relies on individual capacity to exercise agency, rather than ameliorating social causes of illness.

See Chapters 5–7

The trend towards the use of CAM is linked to consumerism and the desire for choice. Easthope (2005) includes providers of complementary health products in a whole new range of industries around consumer choice and the capacity to view health as a product. Other providers in this new way of dealing with the body include the health and beauty industries and the physical fitness and gym industries. The exercise of consumer choice can also be understood as a response to perceived uncertainty in a postmodern society—that is, it reflects a desire to gain control over one's life.

The reasons that CAM use has grown in popularity from the consumer's perspective are encapsulated in this passage from Kaptchuk and Eisenberg (1998: 1062–3):

> The science of complementary medicine, unlike the science component of biomedicine, does not marginalize or deny human experience; rather it affirms patients' real life worlds. When illness (and, sometimes, biomedicine) threatens a patient's capacity for self-knowledge and interpretation, alternative medicine reaffirms the reality of his or her experience.

Question for reflection

What do you think is the most important reason people choose to use CAM?

The convergence of complementary and alternative medicines

Describing CAM as outside the mainstream serves both to differentiate and exclude it from conventional medicine. This section will explore the ways that CAM has converged and become incorporated into orthodox medicine in ways that legitimise its place within the biomedical sphere.

Willis (1994) argues that the similarities in health care practices and the processes of legitimacy are such that all health practices converge into the sphere of health care provision. He provides the following evidence to support his claim that there is a convergence between orthodox and non-orthodox health practices:

- Practitioners of these modalities have gradually and now commonly include components of diagnosis that have techniques common in conventional medical treatment (e.g. take history, blood pressure, physical examination).
- The trend towards recognition of limitations of CAM and thus referral to other practitioners (including orthodox medical practitioners).
- Growing recognition that elements of complementary therapies are also practised by some members of the medical profession. 'The question is not so much the techniques or indeed the paradigms of knowledge themselves, but who should perform them'.
- Recognition that scientific legitimacy is not the only basis for politico-legal legitimation, clinical legitimacy is also important. 'In order to survive and flourish over time any health occupation must continue to be patronised by clients'. (Willis, 1994: 63–4)

There is also a trend towards orthodox medical practice utilising specific therapies in its practice (e.g. acupuncture). This is what is termed incorporation. It is a strategy by which medicine works to remain dominant in the field of health care in the face of increasing numbers of consumers seeking different methods of care. Acupuncture provides an interesting example, where Medicare rebates are now offered if the service is performed by a medical doctor, but not by a qualified acupuncturist. Easthope et al. (1998) report that increasing numbers of general practitioners in Australia are providing acupuncture to their patients. Research by May and Sirur (1998) studied a group of general practitioners in the United Kingdom who incorporated homeopathy into their practice. This study revealed that the appeal of homeopathy lay in its holistic approach. The doctors in the study also believed that homeopathy could do no harm and even without compelling scientific evidence they saw visible results in their patients' recovery.

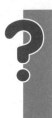

Question for reflection

Are the processes of convergence and incorporation evidence of medical doctors' increased willingness to include alternative therapies to benefit their patients, or are they evidence of medicine's concern with maintaining its occupational territory?

Nurses and complementary and alternative medicine

Tovey and Adams (2003) suggest that nurses are at the forefront of the integration of CAM. They locate the inclusion of CAM into nursing practice in debates about the nature and scope of nursing. Their research has found that incorporating CAM into nursing practice is consistent with the traditional forms of nursing concerned more with individual hands-on care. In addition to this, nursing is also amenable to the innovation and flexibility that come from incorporating CAM into practice. The professional ideology of nursing is such that it is patient-centred, which is also suited to the holistic characteristics of CAM. In this way, they argue that these characteristics of nursing are used to authenticate a role for CAM within nursing.

Similarly, Hansen (2007) suggests that holistic wellness nursing is congruent with the incorporation of CAM. Holistic wellness nursing is described as 'a nursing philosophy that stresses the importance of maintaining health, the "whole person" and self responsibility for health and well-being' (Chambers-Clark, 1986 cited in Hansen, 2007). Its holistic approach is in common with CAM, as is the focus on individual responsibility. This form of nursing practice concerns itself with the maintenance of health and prevention of ill health. Again, another parallel with CAM is that many people use CAM as a way of staying healthy, rather than just something they use when they are ill. While CAM is not essential to holistic or wellness nursing, nurses who identify themselves as holistic or wellness nurses appear more likely to use various types of CAM, such as affirmations, guided imagery, energy healing, acupuncture, aromatherapy and therapeutic massage.

At the end of today's lecture, Julia thinks about the case study that was discussed about the late Jim Bacon and Professor Lowenthal. She reflected on the questions that her lecturers raised about issues of authority and legitimacy, and in particular, she wondered how she would have approached the issue if she, or anyone in her family, was faced with cancer. While she understands that biomedical knowledge dominates the medical profession, Julia still believes that the Director of Medical Oncology at the Royal Hobart Hospital would surely know what he was talking about. Why would anybody question such expertise? But Julia knows that there are other dynamics at play. Some of the questions that may help deconstruct the issues are:

- Why does Lowenthal state a need for 'authoritative evidence-based information'? What type of knowledge does this comment reflect? How does his use of language represent 'authority'?

case study

■ Can you think of some reasons why Jim Bacon received so many pieces of information relating to complementary and alternative therapies? Does this reflect any changes in society's approach to orthodox medicine? Why or why not?

How can Julia think about CAM as an alternative category of health care services? Let's say that Julia was regularly suffering from migraine headaches and that some of the common over-the-counter relief, like Ibuprofen, wasn't effective. There are a lot of pharmaceutical remedies for migraine headaches but many have adverse side effects that Julia would rather not risk; after all, feeling light-headed and drowsy from medication wouldn't assist her in her studies! She looks to a number of alternative health practitioners, and decides to see an acupuncturist and a herbalist. Both practitioners are located at a natural health clinic in her local area and neither has trained as a medical doctor. After a number of visits to the clinic, Julia is feeling a dramatic difference; her headaches are occurring less frequently and are much shorter in duration. She has no side effects from the acupuncture treatment at all, and while the herbs taste unusual, Julia is happy to continue using them as a daily tea tonic. Julia decides that if she ever had a very bad migraine again, she would consult her family doctor, but would continue to use acupuncture and herbal tonics to complement more orthodox treatments.

When Julia visited Medicare to organise payments for her treatments, she was surprised to find that she could not get a rebate for either service. She was told she should have gone to her general practitioner if she wanted to get a rebate for the acupuncture. But how are they different? Julia was obviously aware that both of these treatments were not conventional ways to relieve her migraines, but surely if Julia is experiencing improvements as a result of her chosen therapy, the treatments should be legitimately recognised by the health care system. Julia questions some of the ways in which the health care industry is organised in terms of the legitimacy and authority accorded to particular treatments and therapies, and the type of health care provider.

Questions

1   Why would acupuncture performed by a medical practitioner be viewed as being more legitimate than when performed by a non-medically trained acupuncturist, and why aren't herbalists regarded as health practitioners? Are these issues of authority or legitimacy, or both?

2   Think about scientific and clinical legitimacy. Is it better that people get well after treatment, or that treatments can scientifically prove efficacy? How would you justify your answer?

3   How would you suggest practitioners of CAM improve their legitimacy? Do you think improvements in CAM would necessarily threaten biomedical domination? Why or why not?

CONCLUSION

CAM poses a challenge to a health care system that is based on a biomedical approach. CAM represents a set of ideas about health, some of which may overlap with biomedicine, and some of which may be entirely different. It is important to note from a sociological perspective that one is not better than the other—rather, it is argued that while CAM may be perceived as better because they are holistic, they too do not focus attention on the broader society, often focusing on the individual. A sociological perspective also provides us with an understanding that particular forms of health care and health care practitioners are privileged—that is, they are provided with more legitimacy and power than others.

REVIEW QUESTIONS

1   Why is the quest for legitimacy integral to the acceptance of alternative or complementary healing modalities?

2   How can alternative and complementary healers overcome the tension between their philosophical frameworks on the one hand, and the need for scientific evidence on the other?

3   To what extent are biomedical and CAM philosophies aligned in their emphasis on the individual?

KEY TERMS

Complementary and alternative medicines
Convergence
Incorporation
Legitimacy/legitimation

Medicalisation
Politico-legal, scientific and clinical
      legitimacy

FURTHER READING

Australian Bureau of Statistics 2006, *National Health Survey: Summary of Results*, Canberra, Australian Bureau of Statistics.

Barry, A.M. and Yuill, C. 2002, *Understanding Health: A Sociological Introduction*, London, Sage.

Cant, S. and Sharma, U. (eds) 1996, *Complementary and Alternative Medicines*, London, Free Association Books.

Clavarino, A. and Yates, P. 1995, 'Fear, faith or rational choice: understanding the users of alternative therapies', in Lupton, G. and Najman, J. (eds), *Sociology of Health and Illness: Australian Readings*, Melbourne, Macmillan, pp. 252–75.

Easthope, G. 2005, 'Alternative medicine', in Germov, J. (ed.), *Second Opinion: An Introduction to Health Sociology*, South Melbourne, Oxford University Press.

Hansen, E. 2007, 'CAM, wellness nursing and the new public health', in Adams, J. and Tovey, P. (eds), *Complementary and Alternative Medicine in Nursing and Midwifery: Towards a Critical Social Science*, London, Routledge.

Panel on Definition and Description CRMCA 1997, 'Defining and describing complementary and alternative medicine', *Alternative Therapies*, 3, pp. 49–57.

Saks, M. 2003, *Orthodox and Alternative Medicine*, London, Continuum.

Tovey, P., Easthope, G. and Adams, J. 2004, *The Mainstreaming of Complementary and Alternative Medicine: Studies in Social Context*, London, Routledge.

Willis, E. 1994, *Illness and Social Relations: Issues in the Sociology of Health Care*, St Leonards, Allen & Unwin.

Chapter 13

Nursing in Contemporary Australia

Introduction

Nursing is currently facing complex challenges from many directions. A worldwide shortage of health professionals, including nurses, has created an imperative to examine and improve nurse education, recruitment and retention. The demand for nurses is being driven in part by the increasing rates of chronic disease and the changing demographics within our society. For example, aged care can be described as a burgeoning industry requiring nurses to provide care both in the community and institutional settings. In the broader context of the health care system, the role and scope of nursing practice is changing, particularly in rural areas where the shortage of all health professionals, including nurses, is most acutely felt. At the same time, nursing is grappling with its status as a profession as it experiences tensions between the provision of holistic care and the requirements of being part of a health system that prioritises cost-cutting and efficiency. Taking a sociological perspective to examine these challenges requires consideration of how nursing roles and the scope of practice have changed over time. This helps to analyse the ways that nursing has sought to position itself as a profession and how such positioning is shaped by interactions within nursing itself, with the medical profession and with patients.

Objectives

After reading this chapter, you should be able to:

- explain the shifts that have occurred in nursing practice in Australia and how these impact on contemporary understandings of nursing
- evaluate the differing strategies towards professionalism that have been used to advance nursing as a profession (including 'new nursing')
- critically evaluate the shifts towards greater roles for 'practice nurses' and 'nurse practitioners'.

The nursing workforce

The forces that are shaping nursing are partly demographic and partly related to the changing nature of the health care system. For example, the proportion of Australians aged over 65 years is steadily increasing and as people age, the risk of chronic disease, poor health and disability rises. The increased use and rate of development of health care technologies in the acute care setting has resulted in shorter stays in hospital and the discharge of more complex and sicker patients into the community. This has a twofold effect: nursing care in the hospital is busier because of higher rates of patient turnover, an increased level of dependency during admission and complex technical procedures; and nursing care in the community is also made busier by the increased number of patients who are discharged into the community with complex care needs. Government policies such as 'ageing in place' and deinstitutionalisation have had a significant impact on the community sector. These policies have reversed traditional views that older people and people with physical or intellectual disabilities should be cared for in institutions. In addition to these factors, consumers have become more knowledgeable and their expectations about health care have risen dramatically.

See Chapter 11

The nursing workforce is also shaped by the way that nurses participate in the workforce and the demographics of the workforce itself. Nursing attracts a large number of part-time workers, increasing the total number of nurses required. Further the average age of health care workers is increasing and many nurses are retiring from the workforce. For example, the Australian Institute of Health and Welfare (2001) reported that within the 10 years from 1986 to 1996, the percentage of nurses aged less than 25 years had decreased from 23.3 per cent to 7.7 per cent. In the same period, the proportion of nurses aged over 45 years rose from 17.5 per cent to 30.3 per cent. The average age of nurses is around 40 years, and in some states and specialties it is even older. These characteristics of the nursing profession have resulted in many policy decisions and strategies aimed at improving retention. One example is the provision of re-entry programs for those nurses who have taken time away from nursing work. Current and projected estimates of the shortfall of nurses suggest that up to 13,000 additional nurses will be required by 2010, which equates to a doubling of the current number of graduates from nursing courses (Australian Health Workforce Advisory Committee, 2004). One response has been to commit government funding for an additional 4800 nursing places in Australian universities by 2008.

Nurses have strong employment opportunities because of the labour market's shortage of nurses, and this continues to generate interest in the balance between the supply and demand of nurses. Dockery (2004) points out that the shortage is not limited to Australia, and therefore we need to look beyond the institutional and policy settings to understand why this has occurred. Dockery's (2004: 97) research found that many nurses, particularly younger nurses, were 'disaffected with their careers, particularly with respect to public recognition, pay and further opportunities for education and training'. The factors identified as increasing the likelihood that nurses would stay within the profession were job satisfaction, personal safety and recognition (Dockery, 2004). Whether nursing is encapsulated as a profession or as an occupation is fundamental to such workforce issues.

Question for reflection

What do you think are the most important factors in retaining nurses in the health workforce?

Nursing as a profession

A sociological perspective assists in understanding the debates about occupational territory and the importance of attaining professional status. Professional status is important, as it determines levels of education, pay, autonomy and participation in decision making. Functionalist sociological perspectives of professions provide a framework for understanding how nursing has historically fitted within the health occupational structure. These explanations focus on the contributions that professions make to society through the acquisition of knowledge and skills and commitment to community service, which are rewarded by high earnings and prestige (Wilkinson & Miers, 1999). These theories have been influential in viewing nursing as a semi-profession, largely because it is viewed as not having its own systematic knowledge base and because the work of nurses is subordinated to the medical profession. Wilkinson and Miers (1999: 26) explain that an inherent weakness in these theories is their failure to account for issues of power and control, and as such they served to justify 'the privileged position of specific occupational groups such as doctors and lawyers at a particular historical time'.

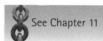
See Chapter 11

Turner's (1987) analysis of professions and the process of professionalisation takes account of the issues relating to power and control. He argues that moves toward professionalisation must be seen as strategies of occupational control—that is, a way for members of an occupation to protect their occupational territory. He proposes three dimensions that need to be considered in examining the process of professionalisation (Turner, 1987: 140). First, there must be the production and maintenance of a body of esoteric knowledge that requires considerable interpretation in its application. This knowledge base is acquired through university training and socialisation within the profession. The body of knowledge utilised in practice must involve interpretation of individual issues/cases, therefore the work of professionals cannot be reduced to a routine practice. If the knowledge base is able to become fragmented and routinised, there is an argument for deprofessionalisation. Second, the profession needs to maintain and cultivate an extensive clientele for its services and this involves various exclusionary practices, whereby competing occupations are subordinated or removed from the marketplace. Finally, a professional group seeks to maintain certain privileges at the point of work and the delivery of a service, namely to maintain autonomy over the delivery of skills and the relationship with the client. Chapter 11 examined the way that the medical profession has successfully used these professionalisation strategies.

See Chapter 11

Another important factor in becoming a profession is the capacity to exercise 'occupational closure'. The concept of occupational closure is based on Weber's idea of social closure, whereby some people are excluded from the membership of status groups. Strategies affecting occupational control include limiting entry to a profession through restricting access to education, training, opportunities and other resources. Achieving occupational closure, however, is not straightforward, as Wilkinson and Miers (1999: 28) explain that 'the process of gaining, retaining and restricting professional skills, knowledge and roles is a highly contested one'. Witz (1992) argues that to fully understand occupational closure, we need to consider the individual, empirical and historical dimensions in which it occurs, as well as the variety of closure practices that professionalising occupations draw upon. Witz (1992) uses the term 'professional project' to denote the historically bounded nature of the professionalising strategies of occupational closure. For example, the 1858 *Medical (Registration) Act* effectively excluded women from the medical profession because, even though it did not explicitly state that women could not be registered, women were excluded from medical education and examination, which were prerequisites for registration. Witz (1992) argues that the creation of a male monopoly within the medical profession is an exemplar of a male professional project.

Professional projects within nursing include strategies for gaining occupational control by demarcating and defending nursing occupational territory (usurpation) and restricting entry into the profession (exclusion). These strategies of usurpation and exclusion are known as dual closure (Witz, 1992). The intended outcome of these strategies is to resist and challenge external control of nursing from the medical profession and hospital authorities, and to establish self-regulation of the nursing profession (Wilkinson & Miers, 1999). The strategies also serve to differentiate clearly between professional nurses and enrolled nurses or health care assistants. In order to examine the implications of professional projects further, it is necessary to describe the history of nursing in Australia, the development of nursing knowledge ('new nursing') and strategies devised to increase the independence and autonomy of nursing.

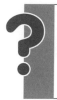

Questions for reflection

Do you think that nursing is viewed as a profession by the general public? Why? Do you think this view is shared by other health professionals?

Early nursing in Australia

The establishment of nursing in Australia was strongly influenced by the country's beginnings as a penal colony. At this time, the primary concern was the development of the colony and, as such, priority was given to building and agriculture, so few resources were devoted, and little credence was paid, to caring for the sick (Cushing, 1997). During early settlement, the majority of health care workers came from convict backgrounds that were considered unsuitable for labouring or other more useful work. Nursing therefore came to be viewed as a role suitable only for those who were socially outcast. As a result, the standard of nursing care was very poor and the nurses themselves were dishevelled, dirty and often intoxicated at work. This time in Australian nursing history is referred to as the 'Dark Age of Nursing' (Schulz, 1991).

As a British colony, Australia's ties to England also proved instrumental in the development of nursing. In the mid 1800s, Florence Nightingale was credited with transforming nursing in England, although some of her critics claim that she took credit for changes that were occurring in the broader social structure (reform of charity) and in the development of medicine (improvement in surgical techniques, hospital reform). In her efforts to change nursing, Nightingale recruited nurses who were more 'middle class' and 'she demanded women who knew their place, were hardworking and uncomplaining and caused no trouble for their employer or supervisor' (George & Davis, 1998: 215). Her view of health and healing is referred to as the sanitarian view, whereby nursing involved control of the environment, through activities such as cleaning, cleanliness and ensuring order so that patients could restore their health (Nelson, 2001). Thus, nurses were expected to be respectable and disciplined, and were readily dismissed if they did not live up to these expectations. Nightingale instutionalised this approach to nursing through the establishment of a nursing school, one of the first steps towards 'modern nursing', although it focused more on the development of the nurse's character than on knowledge and training.

Henry Parkes (the New South Wales Colonial Secretary) invited Florence Nightingale to establish the Nightingale Nursing in Australia in 1866, and in 1868 Lucy Osborn led a team of five Nightingale nurses to Sydney, with the aim of transforming the Sydney Infirmary into a clean and orderly environment

(Godden, 2001). This task was much more difficult than expected. Nelson (2001) describes how Osburn dismissed the worst nurses and then set about reforming the remaining nurses by teaching them hairdressing and issuing uniforms as a first step towards improving their image and decorum. Nelson (2001: 29) argues that in this way 'the professionalisation of nursing, then, was premised upon the grooming and inculcation of desirable virtues into common women'. Nelson (2001) explains that the reshaping of common women working as nurses was not only necessary to reform the hospitals, but also it meant that nurses had to govern themselves (under surveillance and discipline), which in turn gave them the authority to govern and regulate the patients in their care (Nelson, 2001). Osburn experienced difficulty replicating Nightingale Nursing in the colony, particularly with members of her team who assumed moral and social superiority over their colonial counterparts, which resulted in much resentment. In response, Osburn trained many Australian-born as well as British nurses, a move viewed as subversive and autocratic by Florence Nightingale (Godden, 2001). Thus, the establishment of nursing in Australia was influenced by class and existing gender relations, which saw that women's social position was replicated in the workplace through their subservience to the medical profession.

Following the introduction of training for nurses, and the cosmetic changes commenced by Osburn, nursing became a more socially acceptable occupation. As hospital care became safer and more acceptable, the number of hospitals increased and so, too, did the demand for nurses. This in turn, resulted in the need for standardised nurse training and education, and led to the development of registration processes. These registration processes hinged on the need for a set of core skills or competencies that could be examined before admission to the register. The idea of nurse registration was highly contested. Nightingale strongly opposed registration, as her primary concern was with the development of character, which she argued was not examinable (Nelson, 2001). Hospital matrons saw the introduction of registration as reflecting a 'socialist tendency' within nursing and potentially lessening their power (Keleher, 2003). Doctors also opposed registration, fearing that it might lessen their control over nursing (George & Davis, 1998). Nurse registration was legislated in Australia in the 1920s; however, while the register served to distinguish between trained and untrained nurses, it did not achieve the aim of standardising the content or quality of nurse training and education. Nor did it significantly progress nursing towards recognition as a profession, primarily because the hospitals had become firmly entrenched within the health care system and any move to raise hospital education standards was likely to be met with strong opposition because of its impact on resources and workload within the hospital system (Keleher, 2003).

The early attempts at professionalising nursing emulated the masculine approaches of the medical profession, such as credentialing and excluding nonqualified people from nursing practice (Zadoroznyj, 1998). These forms of occupational closure met with limited success because nursing was predominantly female, which meant that nursing was viewed as an extension of 'women's work' and, therefore, the knowledge and skills required were assumed to be minimal. Nurses were also viewed as altruistic and service oriented, so the need for remuneration was assumed to be secondary. It was also difficult for nurses to clearly demarcate their role in relation to other health occupations. Within nursing, the different interests of the groups of nurses also limited the success of these strategies. For example, those from higher social classes sought to exclude women from working-class backgrounds through raising standards (known as the 'professionalisers'), while many nurses were more interested in a job that was well paid rather than an altruistic career (known as the 'unionisers') (George & Davis, 1998). Zadoroznyj (1998: 19) argues that this early approach to professionalisation is criticised because it is 'divisive, elitist, ideologically driven and does not challenge medical dominance in the health care arena'.

By the 1960s, considerable diversification had occurred within nursing. Nurses worked in many different clinical areas and locations. These divisions hampered nurses' ability to mobilise collectively to progress the occupation. During this time, nursing was influenced by factors in the broader social and political arenas, such as the rise of feminism and changing social norms. Nurses became increasingly dissatisfied with their wages and work conditions, and began the process of unionisation. While some considered unionisation as detracting from the ideal of altruistic service, it was an important strategy of occupational closure through tactics of usurpation, such as collective bargaining and labour militancy (Zadoroznyj, 1998). During the 1960s and 1970s, nursing unions grew larger and stronger, and industrial action increased. In 1985, the Royal Australian Nurses Federation removed its long-standing no-strike clause. Unionisation thus profoundly changed nursing and linked professionalisation strategies such as occupational closure with industrial concerns.

Question for reflection

In what ways do you think contemporary nursing reflects its colonial origins?

'New nursing'

In the 1970s, nursing began to develop its own knowledge base, theories and models, arguably the foundations for the 'new nursing'. The development of the nursing process, including the nursing history, assessment and care plan, served to differentiate the work of nurses from the work of doctors and, at the same time, contributed to giving nurses more control over nursing (Wilkinson & Miers, 1999). However, it remains difficult for nursing to establish its own exclusive domain of knowledge, as nursing care is developed, on the one hand, in response to patient needs and, on the other, in conjunction with a knowledge base that is largely shared with doctors and other health care professionals.

The development of nursing theories and models has led to a focus on the content of nursing work. Nursing work became delineated from medicine on the basis of its emphasis on care rather than treatment or cure, and with a holistic approach rather than one that focuses on the disease or illness. Miers (1999: 94) explains that '[e]mphasis on nurses' work outside the medical model has led to an exploration of nursing care as opposed to skills supportive in medical "cure" work'. The development of the nursing process included a nursing approach to patient history taking, diagnosis of nursing problems and the planning of nursing care. These are arguably a nursing response to medicine's monopoly of diagnosis and treatment.

In considering the ways that nursing is differentiated from medicine, attention was drawn to the psycho-social dimensions of nursing, generating discussions about the nature of knowledge and the need for interpretive approaches to knowledge generation in contrast to the positivistic and objective approaches within biomedicine (Degeling et al., 2000). Importantly, these debates led to academic research about the social and interpersonal dimensions of nursing in recognition of the need to incorporate both the patients and the nurses' experience of care (Degeling et al., 2000).

New nursing, as it is known in the United Kingdom, is a professionalising strategy that is 'aimed at carving out an area of functional autonomy in order to augment the status and material rewards of nurses' (Allen, 1997: 502). The new nursing approach is a rejection of the hierarchical and task-focused approach to nursing in favour of the provision of care by professional nurses who take responsibility for individualised whole-of-patient care (Miers, 1999). This is in contrast to team nursing or task nursing, whereby the tasks to be performed during the shift are allocated to various members of the team according to skill level. For example, one nurse may be responsible for all the medications, another for bathing and another for recording patient observations. In the new nursing approach, it is argued that nurses are responsible for a smaller number of patients in a more in-depth and holistic manner, which in turn alters the relationship between nurse–patient (Porter, 1999; Svensson, 1996). Patient participation in their health care is also a characteristic of this approach (Miers, 1999).

The philosophy of the new nursing approach is evident in the changes that have occurred in the last twenty years within nursing in Australia. Wicks (2005) argues that these changes have been most successful when the nursing agenda is congruent with broader political agendas, and provides five examples where this has occurred. First was the move from on-the-job training for nurses to university education, which began in Australia in 1985 in New South Wales. This was an important professional project for nursing; however, its cost-cutting potential had widespread political appeal. The implementation of a career structure for nursing is the second example where new nursing has had an effect by increasing recognition for nurses, in terms of both financial remuneration and occupational status. The establishment of women's health nurses, in New South Wales in 1987, represented a significant move towards nurses practising independently from doctors, including roles in performing diagnostic tests, prescribing and treatment. The fourth example provided by Wicks (2005) is the development of conjoint appointments between teaching hospitals and universities, symbolically and practically bridging the practice-based discipline of nursing with academia. The final example is that of the independent nurse practitioner role (described in detail below).

Question for reflection

How successful do you think nursing has been in differentiating 'nursing care' from the care provided by other health professionals?

Nursing and the medical profession

Classic sociological interpretations of nursing tend to depict nursing rather negatively as a profession that is controlled and dominated by the medical profession (Wicks, 2005). Earlier sociological theories focused on the role of social structure in shaping and controlling nurses' work, identity and behaviour (Wicks, 2005). Gender and class have featured prominently in these accounts. For example, '[t]he power of women as moral forces within the home is argued to have provided the rationale for the extension of this domestic sphere of influence into the public domain … maternal nurturing coupled with domestic organisational skills make the hospital the perfect site for female expertise' (Nelson, 2001: 30). Critiques of the (over)emphasis of gender suggest that these analyses were in a sense 'gender blind'—that is, they have been blind to the professional projects of women because of their focus on the male professional projects, for example, medical dominance (Porter, 1999; Witz, 1992).

Some writers argued that nurses in fact did wield considerable influence in relation to decisions about patient care; however, this influence was exerted subtly and by way of inference rather than in a direct and straightforward manner. This interplay between doctors and nurses became known as the 'doctor–nurse game' (Stein, 1967). More recent analyses, particularly critical and feminist perspectives, have reconsidered the 'traditional' views of nursing as subordinate and revealed how nurses have acted in ways that are contrary and even challenging to those in authority. Porter (1999) suggests that the nurse–doctor power relations can be described in four different ways: nursing as subservient (no/little power), nursing as making hidden recommendations (manipulative power, e.g. the doctor–nurse game, Stein 1967), nursing as making open contributions (cooperative power) and nursing as autonomous (independent power).

There is also a view that the interplay between doctors and nurses is influenced by the broader social context and the situation in which the interactions take place. Svensson (1996: 380) describes this as a negotiated order approach, which refers to the way things get done in organisations as a result of people negotiating with each other. His study of the interplay between nurses and doctors in medical and surgical wards in Sweden found that 'nurses have increased their influence over decisions which affect the patient, and they can influence the norms for interaction and work performance to a greater extent than previously' (Svensson, 1996: 396). He claims that these findings can be explained in the context of changing circumstances within the negotiation context, such as social change and organisational reforms. Others have highlighted ways that doctors and nurses come to work together in a much less competitive and more cooperative way. For example, Carmel's (2006) study of the interaction between doctors and nurses in intensive care units found that the occupational boundaries between the two professions are lessened and the organisational boundaries between the intensive care unit and the rest of the hospital are intensified. Carmel described this as a process of incorporation whereby the doctors and nurses working in the intensive care unit develop a joint perspective.

In light of recent evidence and re-theorising of doctor–nurse interaction, it appears that changing the power balance towards a more egalitarian working relationship may be possible, particularly in clinical settings that enable continuity of staff and specialty—for example, intensive care or accident and emergency departments. These more recent studies of the doctor–nurse interaction shift the focus from social structure (gender and class) towards social theories that allow for the possibility of nurses exercising agency and resistance. While opening up possibilities for change, nursing is still confronted by a health care system and a wider social and political structure that are difficult to change.

Over dinner one night, Julia listens to her mother reminisce about her days as a student nurse within the hospital. Julia's mother spoke of the hierarchy among the nurses on the ward, and the 'unofficial pecking order.' Julia pondered how her encounters with the registered nurses on the wards during practice had been much more collegial, even though she was very much aware of her 'student' status. She was surprised that even nurses who had graduated only one or two years ago seemed to have forgotten what it was like to be a student and assumed the status of an expert. What's more, they seemed to fit right in with the other nurses and doctors. Julia recalled how she had observed nurses making hidden recommendations when interacting with doctors. For example, the nurses didn't ask the doctors to wash their hands in between patients, instead they stated 'Doctor, if you'd like to wash your hands, the sink is over there'. Julia wondered if much had changed in relation to the doctor–nurse game.

Question for reflection

Discuss the ways that the interplay between doctors and nurses reflects the structure–agency debate.

Claims to professionalism: the importance of autonomy

Contemporary nursing theories emphasise nurse autonomy (evidenced by new nursing). The need for autonomy over the provision of care and the patient relationship feature prominently in sociological accounts of the nursing profession that focus less on functionalist accounts and more on understanding nursing's power and status (Degeling et al., 2000). In this section we critically examine the claims to autonomy in nursing practice, by presenting two examples—general practice nurses and nurse practitioners.

General practice nurses

Changes that have occurred within the broader socio-political context of nursing are particularly evident when we examine the role of nurses within general practice. General practice nurses are employed in medical (general) practices to assist general practitioners (GPs) in a range of services—for example, working with patients to improve chronic disease management. Advocates of general practice nurses see them as contributing to improved quality health outcomes, a multidisciplinary approach and bringing specific (specialised) skills to general practice (Royal College of Nursing Australia, 2003). Registered and enrolled nurses in general practice must meet competency standards in addition to the core competencies needed to be registered as a nurse. The scope of practice for nurses in general practice is based on their education, knowledge, competency, experience and lawful authority, and because of this variability, it is suggested that the general practitioner and the nurse negotiate the acceptable scope of practice (Royal College of Nursing Australia, 2003).

Within this clinical area, nurses have gained in both functional autonomy and status, and general practice nursing is now recognised as a specialty area by both nursing and medicine. The developments in this area are further evidence of congruence between political agendas and nursing (Wicks, 2005). The Australian Government has actively supported nurses in general practice and these initiatives have been well received. These include:

- increased funding for practice nursing training and professional support, including funding for practice nurses in rural and remote areas, and in areas of workforce shortage
- Medicare Benefits Schedule items for practice nurses to provide services such as immunisation, wound management and Pap smears
- funding for GPs to be assisted by a practice nurse to manage the health needs of patients with chronic illnesses
- funding for GPs to release practice nurses to attend training on identifying and responding to domestic violence
- a Practice Nurses Scholarship scheme
- funding to develop a national falls prevention and assessment education program for general practice nurses.

The National Practice Nurse Workforce Survey Report (Australian Divisions of General Practice, 2006) reveals that the estimated number of practice nurses has increased by 23 per cent in the past two years to 4924 and, over the same time period, the percentage of general practices that employ one or more nurses has increased by 17 per cent to 57 per cent. As at May 2006, 640 practices were participating in the Practice Incentive Program Urban Practice Nurse Initiative, which is available in urban areas of workforce shortage, and 1100 rural practices were participating in the Practice Incentive Program Rural Nurse Initiative (Australian Government Department of Health and Ageing, 2007b).

Nurses working in general practice have achieved state-sanctioned recognition and legitimacy as evidenced by the substantial injection of funding into this area and the provision of Medicare Benefits Schedule items directly related to nursing care. Pascoe et al. (2005: 44) claim '[i]t appears that nurses working in general practice are no longer the "handmaiden" to the doctor but are professionals who perform a vast range of clinical, administrative and organisational responsibilities within the general practice primary health care setting'. The official documentation about the role of general practice nurses is quite emphatic about their role of working alongside general practitioners and not as a substitute for them. However, in practice it appears that there has been a considerable lag between the implementation of the funding initiatives and the acknowledgment of the importance (specialty) of the general practice nurse role. For example, Watts et al. (2004: xiv) argue that '[t]here is little recognition, acceptance, encouragement, education or support available to build the capacity of nurses to contribute to the future of general practice', with nurses primarily acting as a replacement for overworked GPs.

Nurse practitioners

There are varying definitions of nurse practitioners, but most emphasise advanced educational preparation and experience. 'The nurse practitioner is an extended and advanced practice role of the registered nurse, which may encompass prescribing, diagnosis including the use of diagnostic tests, and referral. The role is characterised by expert clinical knowledge, advanced specialised education and complex decision making skills' (Department of Health and Human Services, 2006). The introduction of the nurse practitioner role in Australia has been prolonged and contested. The first nurse practitioner pilots were implemented, after five years of discussion and planning, in 1995 in New South Wales. A three-year project resulted in the National Competency Standards for the Nurse Practitioner (2006), which specifies the role and scope of nurse practitioners and provides the basis for credentialing and practice standards.

In Australia, the title of 'nurse practitioner' is protected, which means that a registered nurse needs to be authorised by the registration body in their state/territory to call themselves a nurse practitioner. There are a number of steps towards progression to a nurse practitioner:

- gaining undergraduate nursing degree and registration
- post-registration practice progressing to experience at an advanced practice level
- attainment of a required postgraduate educational qualification
- expression of interest in nurse practitioner role
- preparation of an application for recognition as nurse practitioner
- lodging of application and consideration of application by the Board (National Nursing & Nursing Education Taskforce, 2005: 16).

Nurse practitioners in Australia are limited in their scope of practice because of state and territory legislation. For example, nurse practitioners are unable to access the Medical Benefits Scheme or the Pharmaceutical Benefits Scheme. The role of the nurse practitioner has been strongly resisted on the whole by the medical profession. The Australian Medical Association (AMA) initially rejected the principles and roles of nurse practitioners, stating that only medical practitioners could provide comprehensive patient care. Research has found that resistance to the nurse practitioner role by some doctors stems from their concern that they may lose their patients (i.e. their business) (Wilson et al., 2005). This is evident in a joint statement by the New South Wales AMA, the New South Wales faculty of the Royal Australian College of General Practitioners and the Australian College of Rural and Remote Medicine that sought to limit the placement of nurse practitioners to areas 'where there is a locally agreed need and no doctor can be found' (Wicks, 2005: 329). This echoes the previous argument about general practice nurses that nurses are only seen as a suitable substitute for overworked, time-poor or nonexistent doctors.

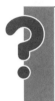

Question for reflection

Compare and contrast the different levels of autonomy afforded to general practice nurses and nurse practitioners.

The nurse–patient relationship

The previous discussion has focused attention on the professionalisation strategies of nursing. Seeking greater legitimacy for nursing as a profession has focused on strategies within nursing, such as occupational closure, and outside the profession, with negotiations to recognise a broader scope of practice for nurses. What must also be examined is how the reshaping of the nursing profession has influenced the relationship between nurses and their patients.

As noted earlier, a key component of being defined as a profession has been the extent to which the service provided is specialised (i.e. not routinised). However, nurses are working in an environment where routinisation may in fact be beneficial, in that clearly defined clinical pathways for various conditions that map out the expected events in a patient's recovery may extend nursing autonomy. This must be balanced alongside the emphasis in new nursing on patient care being individualised, and where the uniqueness of the individual is emphasised. Degeling et al. (2000: 127) argue that nurses prefer decision-making processes that are not only guided by rules, but also 'defer to custom and precedent rather than formal rationality'. With reference to Turner's (1987) description of the dimensions of professions, this resistance can be understood as protection against the deprofessionalisation that may occur if nursing work becomes routine and fragmented or the need for interpretation of individual cases is no longer required. Malone (2003) also argues that the standardisation of care and introduction of structured forms of charting patient care result in a loss of physical proximity with the patient. She refers to this as 'distal nursing',

See Chapter 11

which is a 'highly rationalised, abstract representation of what nurses do that makes perfect sense within a perspective distant from actual care situations' (Malone, 2003: 2323).

Nurses are depicted within the nursing literature as central to the management of patient care. This indicates that there has been a shift from positioning nurses as the 'doctor's handmaiden' to the position of 'physician's complement' (Degeling et al., 2000). A small study conducted in Queensland about women's views of registered nurses as Pap smear providers suggests that the substitution of doctors by nurses in this instance was well accepted (Christie et al., 2005). Another study of the acceptance of nurses within general practice found that consumers 'accepted this new role because they trusted the doctor to employ suitably qualified and competent nurses and they expected that doctors and practice nurses would work collaboratively and in the best interests of the consumer' (Hegney et al., 2006: 49). Thus, in this instance, it would appear the acceptance of the nurses is more related to the trust and credibility of the doctor than the nurses themselves.

The changing position of nurses in relation to doctors in the management of care is also evident in the description of the nurse–patient relationship as a partnership in which the nurse 'moves from being an expert care provider to being a partner with the client in order to improve the client's capabilities' (Gallant et al., 2002). This shift can be understood in the broader social and political context where there has been a move towards enabling, empowerment and capacity-building strategies, as well as the influence of the consumer movement. This type of relationship is evident in the nursing care of people with a chronic illness. For example, recent research about patients involved with a nurse-led model of care for diabetes experienced shared decision making within the nurse–patient relationship and were found to develop autonomy as a result of the nurses' focus on their individual needs (Moser et al., 2006).

Nursing's knowledge and understanding of the patient influences the way that nurses are positioned in relation to other nurses, other health care providers and the patient. For example, the nurse is simultaneously an advocate, caring supporter and a nurse, among other subject positions that may change according to circumstances, but this can result in internal conflict (Fahy & Smith, 1999). Carroll and Reiger (2005) argue that lactation consultants find themselves in roles that are in conflict between the professional and anti-professional. Their roles are professional because of their formal qualifications and, at the same time, they resist professionalism because they need to give credence to the lived experience of the breastfeeding mothers they are working with. This conflict is also influenced by the need for lactation consultants to establish legitimacy among other health professionals and the ideology of maternalism that underpinned the establishment of these roles. Child health nurses also face similar issues.

Technology has transformed contemporary health care. Often the relationship between nursing and technology is depicted as part of normal care routines and in this way, technology is viewed as neutral. However, as we saw in Chapter 10, sociologists argue that social processes are embedded within technologies that shape its use and its value. Henderson (2006) explains that nursing expertise is legitimised through nurses' knowledge and understanding of the individual and that the expert nurse must take account of technology, but must care for the patient. In the process of catering for the technology, the patient may become invisible, particularly for inexperienced nurses. Henderson (2006: 64) argues that nursing needs to keep sight of the primacy of the patient and to 'shift the social, organisational, political systems so that the power of nursing relationships in the technological environment is based on … shaping the context of care so as to enable ideal practice'.

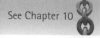
See Chapter 10

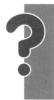

Questions for reflection

Based on the discussion above, which factors do you think are most influential in shaping nursing practice? Why?

CONCLUSION

The professionalising project of nursing provides an excellent case study of occupations and professions in health. There is a need to understand the historical dimensions that relate to issues such as social class and gender, the relationships with other occupations and professions in the health arena, and the competing priorities and strategies that exist within nursing itself. The case examples of practice nurses and nurse practitioners are illustrative of these tensions and contradictions. While taking account of the social and historical contexts, a sociological analysis of occupational territory highlights the capacity of the health workforce to claim legitimacy for work practices, to implement strategies relating to power and control, and to respond to competing demands in an increasingly complex working environment.

REVIEW QUESTIONS

1   How has the historical context of the provision of health care impacted on the development of nursing as a profession?
2   Which strategies of occupational closure have been used most effectively by the nursing profession?

3   How do initiatives such as 'practice nurses' and 'nurse practitioners' challenge medical dominance?

KEY TERMS

Exclusion
New nursing
Occupational closure
Professional project

Professionalisation
Registration
Usurpation

FURTHER READING

Australian Government Department of Health and Ageing 2007a, 'Nursing in general practice', www.health.gov.au/internet/wcms/publishing.nsf/Content/pcd-nursing-index, accessed January 2007.

Australian Health Workforce Advisory Committee 2004, *Annual Report 2003–2004*, Report 2004.3, Sydney, Australian Health Workforce Advisory Committee.

Carmel, S. 2006, 'Health care practices, professions and perspectives: a case study in intensive care', *Social Science & Medicine*, 62, pp. 2079–90.

Christie, L., Gamble, J. and Creedy, D. 2005, 'Women's views of registered nurses as Papanicolaou smear providers: a pilot study', *Contemporary Nurse*, 20, pp. 159–68.

Gallant, M.H., Beaulieu, M.C. and Carnevale, F.A. 2002, 'Partnership: an analysis of the concept within the nurse–client relationship', *Journal of Advanced Nursing*, 40, pp. 149–57.

George, J. and Davis, A. 1998, *States of Health: Health and Illness in Australia*, South Melbourne, Longman.

Hegney, D., Eley, R., Buikstra, E., Rees, S. and Patterson, E. 2006, 'Consumers' level of comfort with an advanced practice role for registered nurses in general practice: a Queensland, Australia, study', *Australian Journal of Primary Health*, 12, pp. 44–51.

Henderson, A. 2006, 'The evolving relationship of technology and nursing practice: negotiating the provision of care in a high tech environment', *Contemporary Nurse*, 22, pp. 59–65.

Keleher, H. 2003, 'Public health nursing in Australia: historically invisible', *International History of Nursing Journal*, 7, pp. 50–5.

Wilkinson, G. and Miers, M. (eds) 1999, *Power and Nursing Practice*, London, Macmillan.

Witz, A. 1992, *Professions and Patriarchy*, London, Routledge.

Chapter 14

Nurses, Sociology and Health

Julia and her mother were once again discussing the pros and cons of university education for nurses. However, this time, it was Julia who had stories to tell. She explained to her mother that she now understood that people experience health and illness differently as a result of their social location, as well as their values and beliefs. Julia talked about how she no longer saw problems such as work accidents, domestic violence and refugee mental health as the private troubles of individuals, but as public issues influenced by broader social forces. Julia's mother was fascinated as she heard Julia recount her newfound understanding of these issues and as she started to reflect on her own understandings, she wondered if there was some merit to this alternative point of view. She suggested to Julia that this was all well and good to know about these types of social issues, but how did this impact on nursing care? Julia recalled examples of the ways that people experience disability and chronic illnesses, such as mental illness, and explained to her mother that this helped her to see the social implications of these conditions. Julia told her mother she truly believed that she would be a better nurse as a result of this knowledge.

In the days following this conversation, Julia's mother began to recall patients that she had looked after and began to see things differently. She remembered a young mother who visited the accident and emergency department on at least three occasions with bruising and lacerations that needing stitching. She suspected at the time that this woman might have been experiencing domestic violence, but she couldn't understand why the woman never left her husband or told anyone what really happened. Julia's mother shuddered as she remembered the mangled state of one young man who had been involved in a single vehicle accident—was it an accident or was it really a suicide attempt? As a community nurse, Julia's mother wondered why people with disabilities or with emphysema didn't get out in the community more but she never fully appreciated how difficult this might have been, nor had she accounted for the stigma associated with 'being different'. When involved in health promotion, Julia's mother couldn't understand why some people never changed their behaviour—maybe it was something to do with the social factors Julia had been talking about. She had also seen this type of non-compliance in her last job working in a general practice surgery, even though when she worked there she was more like a medical receptionist than doing the full range of tasks that nurses currently undertake in general practice. She felt reassured that if Julia was right, she would be a better nurse and be better equipped to deal with the way health needs and the health system have changed.

Sociology is the study of society. In this text, we have presented a broad range of topics to demonstrate its applicability to macro and micro perspectives. By taking a macro perspective, we applied a structural analysis to society to examine the influence of social structures on health. In this way, we highlighted the social determinants of health and how health and illness are socially produced and distributed. Micro perspectives were used to gain a deeper understanding of the experiences of health and illness, and the ways in which these experiences are shaped by societal values and beliefs.

For nurses to function effectively within the health care system they need to understand the social context in which they are operating and how the people they will be caring for construct meanings of health and illness. This book has shown how sociological analyses add to our knowledge of both the social context that nurses work within and that of the people with whom they work and care for. In particular, we have drawn attention to the power relations involved in these interactions.

The topics covered in this book are relevant to all of the aspects of nursing encapsulated in this definition from the International Council of Nurses:

> Nursing encompasses autonomous and collaborative care of individuals of all ages, families, groups and communities, sick or well and in all settings. Nursing includes the promotion of health, prevention of illness, and the care of ill, disabled and dying people. Advocacy, promotion of a safe environment, research, participation in shaping health policy and in patient and health systems management, and education are also key nursing roles. (International Council of Nurses 2007)

The definition above indicates that nursing revolves around social interactions; nurses can develop a more in-depth understanding of these interactions by using the explanatory models offered by sociology. Equipped with a sociological imagination, nurses will have a more informed approach to the provision of care.

We have promoted a critical approach in this text, one that is reflective and questioning. Learning to see things differently, to unpack our taken-for-granted understandings of health and illness and how people experience them is evidence of this. We argue that sociological knowledge also needs to be useful. We agree with Williams, Cooke and May (1998) that sociology is an ethical discipline because it contributes to advocacy as well as understanding. It is not enough that Julia and her fellow nursing students develop a better understanding of issues such as the health of Aboriginal and Torres Strait Islander peoples. They must develop the capacity to incorporate this knowledge into their everyday practice, thereby becoming effective and ethical advocates for the people with whom they work.

references

Abercrombie, N., Hill, S. and Turner, B.S. 2000, *The Penguin Dictionary of Sociology*, London, Penguin.

Aboriginal and Torres Strait Islander Commission 1999, *As Matter of Fact: Answering the Myths and Misconceptions about Indigenous Australians* (3rd edn), Canberra, Commonwealth of Australia.

Adams, J., Sibbritt, D.W., Easthope, G. and Young, A.F. 2003, 'The profile of women who consult alternative health practitioners in Australia', *Medical Journal of Australia*, 179, pp. 297–300.

Ahn, A., Tewari, M., Poon, C.-S. and Phillips, R. 2006, 'The clinical applications of a systems approach', *PLoS Medicine*, 3, 7, pp. 956–60.

Allen, D. 1997, 'The nursing–medical boundary: a negotiated order?', *Sociology of Health and Illness*, 19, 4, pp. 498–520.

Allsop, J. 2006, 'Regaining trust in medicine: professional and state strategies', *Current Sociology*, 54, 4, pp. 621–36.

Alston, M. 2006, ' "I'd like to just walk out of here": Australian women's experience of drought', *Sociologica Ruralis*, 46, 2, pp. 154–70.

Anderson, I. 2004, 'Aboriginal health', in Grbich, C. (ed.), *Health in Australia: Sociological Concepts and Issues* (3rd edn), Frenchs Forest, Pearson Education, pp. 75–100.

Arber, S., McKinlay, J., Adams, A., Marceau, L., Link, C. and O'Donnell, A. 2006, 'Patient characteristics and inequalities in doctors' diagnostic and management strategies relating to CHD: A video-stimulation experiment', *Social Science & Medicine*, 62, 1, pp. 103–15.

Aroni, R., de Boer, R. and Harvey, K. 2003, 'The Viagra affair: evidence as the terrain for competing "partners"', in Lin, V. and Gibson, B. (eds), *Evidence-based Health Policy: Problems and Possibilities*, South Melbourne, Oxford University Press, pp. 97–109.

Australian Bureau of Statistics 2000, 'Work-related injuries, Australia', in *Labour Force, Australia*, Canberra, Australian Bureau of Statistics.

Australian Bureau of Statistics 2003, *Australian Demographic Statistics Quarterly: September Quarter, 2002*, Canberra, Australian Bureau of Statistics.

Australian Bureau of Statistics 2004a, *Migration Australia*, cat. no. 3412.0, Canberra, Australian Government.

Australian Bureau of Statistics 2004b, *Year Book of Australia 2004*, cat. no. 1301.0, Canberra, Australian Bureau of Statistics.

Australian Bureau of Statistics 2004c, *Experimented Estimates and Projections, Aboriginal and Torres Strait Islander Australians 1991 to 1996*, cat. no. 3238.0, Canberra, Australian Bureau of Statistics.

Australian Bureau of Statistics 2006, *National Health Survey: Summary of Results*, Canberra, Australian Bureau of Statistics.

Australian Communications and Media Authority 2006, *About the ACMA*, www.acma.gov.au, accessed 1 June 2006.

Australian Divisions of General Practice (ADGP) 2006, *National Practice Nurse Workforce Survey Report*, Canberra, Australian Government Department of Health and Ageing.

Australian Government Department of Health and Ageing 2006a, *Medicare Funding of Magnetic Radio Imaging at Sydney's Children's Hospital*, Press Release October 2006, www.health.gov.au/internet/ministers/publishing.nsf/Content/health-mediarel-yr2006-ta-abb120.htm?OpenDocument&yr=2006&mth=8

Australian Government Department of Health and Ageing 2006b, *Funding of Herceptin through the Pharmaceutical Benefits Scheme*, Press Release August 2006, www.health.gov.au/internet/ministers/publishing.nsf/Content/health-mediarel-yr2006-ta-abb135.htm?OpenDocument&yr=2006&mth=10

Australian Government Department of Health and Ageing 2007a, *Nursing in General Practice*, www.health.gov.au/internet/wcms/publishing.nsf/Content/pcd-nursing-index, accessed January 2007.

Australian Government Department of Health and Ageing 2007b, *Medicare Australia*, www.medicareaustralia.gov.au, accessed February 2007.

Australian Health Workforce Advisory Committee 2004, *Annual Report 2003–2004*, Report 2004.3, Sydney, Australian Health Workforce Advisory Committee.

Australian Institute of Health and Welfare 2000, *Australia's Health 2000: The Seventh Biennial Health Report of the Australian Institute of Health and Welfare*, Canberra, Australian Institute of Health and Welfare.

Australian Institute of Health and Welfare 2001, 'Nursing Labour Force 1999. AIHW cat. no. HWL 20', in *National Health Labour Force Series No. 20*, Canberra, Australian Institute of Health and Welfare.

Australian Institute of Health and Welfare 2002, *Chronic Diseases and Associated Risk Factors in Australia*, Canberra, Australian Institute of Health and Welfare.

Australian Institute of Health and Welfare 2006, *Australia's Health 2006: The Tenth Biennial Health Report of the Australian Institute of Health and Welfare*, Australian Institute of Health and Welfare, Canberra.

Australian Institute of Health and Welfare: Singh, M. and de Looper, M. 2002, 'Australian health inequalities: 1 birthplace', *Bulletin no. 2*, Canberra, Australian Institute of Health and Welfare.

Australians for Native Title and Reconciliation 2004, *Healing Hands: Indigenous Health Rights Action Kit*, Rozelle, ANTaR.

Backett-Milburn, K., Willis, W., Gregory, S. and Lawton, J. 2006, 'Making sense of eating, weight and risk in the early teenage years: views and concerns of parents in poorer socio-economic circumstances', *Social Science & Medicine*, 63, pp. 624–35.

Baer, H. 2006, 'The drive for legitimation in Australian naturopathy: success and dilemmas', *Social Science & Medicine*, 63, pp. 1771–83.

Bakx, K. 1991, 'The eclipse of folk medicine in western society', *Sociology of Health and Illness*, 13, 1, pp. 20–38.

Barr, T. 2000, *Newsmedia.com.au: The Changing Face of Australia's Media and Communications*, St Leonards, Allen & Unwin.

Barry, A.-M. and Yuill, C. 2002, *Understanding Health: A Sociological Introduction*, London, Sage.

Barry, C.A. 2006, 'The role of evidence in alternative medicine: contrasting bio-medical and anthropological approaches', *Social Science & Medicine*, 62, pp. 2646–57.

Bassett, K., Iyer, N. and Kazanjian, A. 2000, 'Defensive medicine during the hospital obstetric care: a byproduct of the technological age', *Social Science & Medicine*, 51, pp. 523–37.

Baum, F. 2002, *The New Public Health* (2nd edn), South Melbourne, Oxford University Press.

Beck, U. 1992, *Risk Society: Towards a New Modernity*, London, Sage Publications.

Becker, H. 1963, *Outsiders*, New York, Free Press.

Belcher, H. 2005, 'Power, politics and health care', in Germov, J. (ed.), *Second Opinion: An Introduction to Health Sociology*, South Melbourne, Oxford University Press, pp. 267–89.

Bellamy, S. 2005, 'Lives to save lives: the ethics of tissue typing', *Human Fertility*, 8, 1, pp. 5–11.

Bensoussan, A. and Lewith, G.T. 2004, 'Complementary medicine research in Australia: a strategy for the future', *Medical Journal of Australia*, 181, 6, pp. 331–3.

Berger, P.L. and Luckmann, T. 1971, *The Social Construction of Reality*, Harmondsworth, Penguin.

Bickerstaff, H., Finter, F., Toh Yeong, C. and Braude, P. 2001, 'Clinical application of preimplantation genetic diagnosis', *Human Fertility*, 4, pp. 24–30.

Bilton, T., Bonnett, K., Jones, P., Skinner, D., Stanworth, M. and Webster, A. 1996, *Introductory Sociology* (3rd edn), London, Palgrave Macmillan.

Bird, C.E. and Rieker, P.B. 1999, 'Gender matters: an integrated model for understanding men's and women's health', *Social Science & Medicine*, 48, pp. 745–55.

Blane, D. 1985, 'An assessment of the Black Report's "explanations of health inequalities"', *Sociology of Health and Illness*, 7, 3, pp. 423–47.

Bolam, B., Hodgetts, D., Chamberlain, K., Murphy, S. and Gleeson, K. 2003, ' "Just do it": an analysis of accounts of control over health amongst lower socio-economic status groups', *Critical Public Health*, 13, 1, pp. 15–31.

Bordo, S. 1993, *Unbearable Weight: Feminism, Western Culture and the Body*, Berkeley, University of California Press.

Bourdieu, P. 1984, *Distinction: A Social Critique of the Judgement of Taste*, London, Routledge and Kegan Paul.

Brady, M. 1992, *Heavy Metal: The Social Meaning of Petrol Sniffing in Australia*, Canberra, Aboriginal Studies Press.

Brady, M. 2004, *Indigenous Australia and Alcohol Policy: Meeting Difference with Indifference*, Sydney, University of New South Wales Press.

Braude, P., Pickering, S., Flinter, F. and Mackie Olgivie, C. 2002, 'Preimplantation genetic diagnosis', *Nature Reviews*, 3, pp. 941–53.

Brotherhood of St Laurence 2002, 'Seeking asylum: living with fear, uncertainty and exclusion', *Changing Pressures*, Bulletin 11.

Bula Ngumbaay Aboriginal Consultants 2002, *Walking Together: A Toolkit for Working with Aboriginal Communities on the Central Coast of NSW*, Gosford, Central Coast Neighbourhood and Community Centres.

Burdekin, B. 1989, *Our Homeless Children*, Canberra, Human Rights and Equal Opportunities Commission.

Burstein, M. 2005, 'Combating the social exclusion of at-risk groups', Policy Research Initiative Paper, Government of Canada.

Bury, M. 1982, 'Chronic illness as biographical disruption', *Sociology of Health and Illness*, 4, 2, pp. 167–82.

Butler, A. 2002, *Consumer Participation in Australian Primary Care: A Literature Review*, Melbourne, National Resource Centre for Consumer Participation in Health.

Butler, C., Rissel, C. and Khavarpour, F. 1999, 'The context for community participation in health action in Australia', *Australian Journal of Social Issues*, 34, 3, pp. 253–64.

Bytheway, B. and Johnson, J. 1998, 'The sight of age', in Nettleton, S. and Watson, J. (eds), *The Body in Everyday Life*, London, Routledge, pp. 243–57.

Calnan, M. 1987, *Health and Illness: A Lay Perspective*, London, Tavistock.

Cameron, C. and Williamson, R. 2003, 'Is there an ethical difference between pre-implantation genetic diagnosis and abortion?', *Journal of Medical Ethics*, 29, pp. 90–2.

Cameron, P., Willis, K., Western, M. and Jones, G. 2000, *Unemployment and Health*, Burnie, North West Tasmania Division of General Practice.

Cant, S. 1996, 'From charismatic teaching to professional training: the legitimation of knowledge and the creation of trust in homeopathy and chiropractic', in Cant, S. and Sharma, U. (eds), *Complementary and Alternative Medicines*, London, Free Association Books, pp. 44–65.

Cant, S. and Sharma, U. (eds) 1996, *Complementary and Alternative Medicines*, London, Free Association Books.

Carmel, S. 2006, 'Health care practices, professions and perspectives: a case study in intensive care', *Social Science & Medicine*, 62, pp. 2079–90.

Carroll, K. and Reiger, K. 2005, 'Fluid experts: lactation consultants as postmodern professional specialists', *Health Sociology Review*, 14, 2, pp. 101–10.

Carter, M., Walker, C. and Furler, J. 2002, 'Developing a shared definition of chronic illness: the implications and benefits for general practice', www.chronicillness.org.au, accessed 22 September 2006.

Castells, M. 2002, 'The Internet and the network society: series editor's preface', in Wellman, B. and Haythornthwaite, C. (eds), *The Internet in Everyday Life*, Oxford, Blackwell, pp. xxix–xxxi.

Chamberlin, C. and Robinson, P. 2002, *The Needs of Older Gay, Lesbian and Transgender People*, Melbourne, ALSO Foundation.

Chapman, E. 2000, 'Conceptualisation of the body for people living with HIV: issues of touch and examination', *Sociology of Health and Illness*, 22, 6, pp. 840–57.

Cheek, J., Shoebridge, J., Willis, E. and Zadoroznyj, M. 1996, *Society and Health*, Melbourne, Longman.

Christie, L., Gamble, J. and Creedy, D. 2005, 'Women's views of registered nurses as Papanicolaou smear providers: a pilot study', *Contemporary Nurse*, 20, pp. 159–68.

Chronic Illness Alliance 2006, 'Homepage', www.chronicillness.org.au, accessed 22 September 2006.

Clark, R.A., McLennan, S., Eckert, K., Dawson, A., Wilkinson, D. and Stewart, S. 2005, 'Chronic heart failure beyond city limits', *Rural and Remote Health*, 5, p. 443.

Clavarino, A. and Yates, P. 1995, 'Fear, faith or rational choice: understanding the users of alternative therapies', in Lupton, D. and Najman, J. (eds), *Sociology of Health and Illness: Australian Readings*, Melbourne, Macmillan, pp. 252–75.

Collinson, J.A. 2005, 'Emotions, interaction and the injured sporting body', *International Review for the Sociology of Sport*, 40, 2, pp. 221–40.

Collyer, F. 1999, 'The social production of medical technology', in Grbich, C. (ed.), *Health in Australia: Sociological Concepts and Issues* (2nd edn), Frenchs Forest, Pearson, pp. 217–37.

Collyer, F. 2004, 'Medical technology: from drugs to genetics', in Grbich, C. (ed.), *Health in Australia: Sociological Concepts and Issues* (3rd edn), Frenchs Forest, Pearson, pp. 46–72.

Coney, S. 1993, *The Menopause Industry: A Guide to Medicine's 'Discovery' of the Midlife Woman*, North Melbourne, Spinifex.

Connell, R.W. 2005, *Masculinities* (2nd edn), Crows Nest, Allen & Unwin.

Connor, L.H. 2004, 'Relief, risk and renewal; mixed therapy regimens in an Australian suburb', *Social Science & Medicine*, 59, pp. 1695–705.

Conrad, P. 1992, 'Medicalisation and social control', *Annual Review of Sociology*, 18, pp. 209–32.

Conrad, P. 1994, 'Wellness as a virtue: morality and the pursuit of health', *Culture, Medicine & Psychiatry*, 18, pp. 385–401.

Conrad, P. 1998, 'A mirage of genes', *Sociology of Health and Illness*, 21, pp. 228–41.

Corbin, J.M. and Strauss, A. 1988, *Unending Work and Care: Managing Chronic Illness at Home*, San Francisco, Jossey Bass.

Courtenay, W.H. 2000, 'Constructions of masculinity and their influence on men's wellbeing: a theory of gender and health', *Social Science & Medicine*, 50, 10, pp. 1385–401.

Craig, D. 2000, 'Practical logics: the shapes and lessons of popular medical knowledge and practice: examples from Vietnam and Indigenous Australia', *Social Science & Medicine*, 51, pp. 703–11.

Cushing, A. 1997, 'Convicts and care giving in colonial Australia, 1788–1868', in Rafferty, A.M., Robinson, J. and Elkan, R. (eds), *Nursing and the Politics of Welfare*, London, Routledge, pp. 108–32.

Daly, J. 2005, *Evidence-based Medicine and the Search for a Science of Clinical Care*, Berkeley, University of California Press/Milbank Memorial Fund.

Daly, J. and McDonald, I. 1997, 'Cardiac disease construction on the borderland', *Social Science & Medicine*, 44, 7, pp. 1043–9.

David, M. and Kirkhope, J. 2005, 'Cloning/stem cells and the meaning of life', *Current Sociology*, 53, 2, pp. 367–81.

Davis, A. and George, J. 1993, *States of Health: Health and Illness in Australia* (2nd edn), Sydney, Harper Educational.

Davison, C., Frankel, S. and Davey Smith, G. 1992, 'The limits of lifestyle: re-assessing "fatalism" in the popular culture of illness prevention', *Social Science & Medicine*, 34, 6, pp. 675–85.

Degeling, P., Hill, M., Kennedy, J., Coyle, B. and Maxwell, S. 2000, 'A cross-national study of differences in the identities of nursing in England and Australia and how this has affected nurses' capacity to respond to hospital reform', *Nursing Inquiry*, 7, pp. 120–35.

Denton, M., Prus, S. and Walters, V. 2004, 'Gender differences in health: a Canadian study of the psychological, structural and behavioural determinants of health', *Social Science & Medicine*, 58, pp. 2585–600.

Department of Health and Aged Care 1999, 'An overview of health status, health care and public health in Australia', *Department of Health and Aged Care Occasional Papers Series No. 5*, Canberra, Australian Government Department of Health and Aged Care.

Department of Health and Human Services 2006, 'Nurse Practitioner Scoping Project', www.dhhs.tas.gov.au/agency/pro/nursepractitioner/, accessed 13 November 2006.

Dixon, J. and Welch, N. 2000, 'Researching the rural–metropolitan health differential using the "social determinants of health"', *Australian Journal of Rural Health*, 8, pp. 254–60.

Dockery, A.M. 2004, 'Workforce experience and retention in nursing in Australia', *Australian Bulletin of Labour*, 30, 2, pp. 74–100.

Dodson, M. 1993, *Aboriginal and Torres Strait Islander Social Justice Commission First Report 1993*, Canberra, Reconciliation and Social Justice Library, www.austlii.edu.au/au/special/rsjproject/rsjlibrary/hreoc/atsisjc_1993/.

Doran, E., Kerridge, I., McNeill, P. and Henry, D. 2006, 'Empirical uncertainty and moral contest: a qualitative analysis of the relationship between medical specialists and the pharmaceutical industry in Australia', *Social Science & Medicine*, 62, pp. 1510–19.

Doyal, L. 1995, *What Makes Women Sick: Gender and the Political Economy of Health*, Houndmills, Macmillan.

Driscoll, T. and Mayhew, C. 1999, 'Extent and cost of occupational injury and illness', in Mayhew, C. and Peterson, L. (eds), *Occupational Health and Safety in Australia*, Sydney, Allen & Unwin, pp. 28–51.

Durkheim, E. 1970, *Suicide: A Study in Sociology*, London, Routledge & Keegan Paul.

Easthope, G. 2005, 'Alternative medicine', in Germov, J. (ed.), *Second Opinion: An Introduction to Health Sociology* (3rd edn), South Melbourne, Oxford University Press, pp. 332–48.

Easthope, G., Beilby, J.J., Gill, G.F. and Tranter, B.K. 1998, 'Acupuncture in Australian general practice: practitioner characteristics', *Medical Journal of Australia*, 169, pp. 197–200.

Eastwood, H. 2000, 'Why are Australian GPs using alternative medicine? Postmodernisation, consumerism and the shift towards holistic health', *Journal of Sociology*, 36, 2, pp. 133–56.

Ehrenreich, B. and English, D. 1978, 'The "sick" women of the upper classes', in Ehrenreich, J. (ed.), *The Cultural Crisis of Modern Medicine*, New York, Monthly Review Press, pp. 123–43.

Emslie, C., Ridge, D., Ziebland, S. and Hunt, K. 2006, 'Men's accounts of depression: reconstructing or resisting hegemonic masculinity?', *Social Science & Medicine*, 62, 9, pp. 2246–57.

Engels, F. 1845, *The Condition of the Working Class in England*, www.marxists.org/archive/marx/works/1845/condition-working-class/.

Ensign, J. and Panke, E. 2002, 'Barriers and bridges to care: voices of homeless female adolescent youth in Seattle, Washington, USA', *Journal of Advanced Nursing*, 37, 2, pp. 166–72.

Evetts, J. 2006, 'Short note: the sociology of professional groups', *Current Sociology*, 54, 1, pp. 133–43.

Expert Committee on Complementary Medicines in the Health System 2003, *Complementary Medicines in the Australian Health System*, a report to the Parliamentary Secretary to the Minister for Health and Ageing, Commonwealth of Australia.

Ezzy, D. 2000, 'Illness narratives: time, hope and HIV', *Social Science & Medicine*, 50, pp. 387–96.

Fahy, K. and Smith, P. 1999, 'From the sick role to subject positions: a new approach to the medical encounter', *Health*, 3, 1, pp. 71–93.

Financing and Analysis Branch 2000, *The Australian Health Care System: An Outline*, Canberra, Commonwealth Department of Health and Aged Care.

Forbes, A. and Wainwright, S. 2001, 'On the methodological, theoretical and philosophical context of health inequalities research: a critique', *Social Science & Medicine*, 53, pp. 801–16.

Foucault, M. 1973, *Birth of the Clinic: An Archaeology of Medical Perception*, London, Tavistock Publications.

Foucault, M. 1977, *Discipline and Punish: The Birth of the Prison*, London, Penguin Books.

Foucault, M. 1980, 'The eye of power', in Gordon, C. (ed.), *Power/Knowledge: Selected Interviews and Other Writings 1972–1977*, London, Harvester, pp. 146–65.

Fox, R. 1957, 'Training for uncertainty', in Merton, R.K., Reader, G.G. and Kendall, P. (eds), *The Student-Physician*, Cambridge, Harvard University Press.

Frankel, S., Davison, C. and Davey Smith, G. 1991, 'Lay epidemiology and the rationality of responses to health education', *British Journal of General Practice*, 41, pp. 428–30.

Friedson, E. 1970, *The Profession of Medicine*, New York, Dodd Mead.

Furnham, A. 1994, 'Explaining health and illness: lay perceptions on current and future health, the causes of illness and the nature of recovery', *Social Science & Medicine*, 39, 5, pp. 715–25.

Gallant, M.H., Beaulieu, M.C. and Carnevale, F.A. 2002, 'Partnership: an analysis of the concept within the nurse–client relationship', *Journal of Advanced Nursing*, 40, 2, pp. 149–57.

Gavaghan, C. 2003, 'Use of preimplantation diagnosis to produce tissue donors: an irreconcilable dichotomy', *Human Fertility*, 6, pp. 23–5.

Gelijns, A. and Rosenberg, N. 1994, 'The dynamics of technological change in medicine', *Health Affairs*, 13, 3, pp. 28–46.

George, J. and Davis, A. 1998, *States of Health: Health and Illness in Australia* (3rd edn), South Melbourne, Longman.

Germov, J. 1998, 'Glossary', in Germov, J. (ed.), *Second Opinion: An Introduction to Health Sociology*, South Melbourne, Oxford University Press.

Germov, J. 2005, 'Challenges to medical dominance', in Germov, J. (ed.), *Second Opinion: An Introduction to Health Sociology* (3rd edn), South Melbourne, Oxford University Press, pp. 290–313.

Giddens, A. 1991, *Modernity and Self-identity: Self and Society in the Late Modern Age*, Cambridge, Polity.

Gilding, M. 2002, 'Families of the new millenium: designer babies, cyber sex and virtual communities', *Family Matters*, 62, Winter, pp. 4–10.

Gill, R., Henwood, K. and McLean, C. 2005, 'Body projects and the regulation of normative masculinity', *Body & Society*, 11, 1, pp. 37–62.

Gillett, J. 2004, 'Media activism and Internet use by people with HIV/AIDS', in Seale, C. (ed.), *Health and the Media*, Oxford, Blackwell.

Godden, J. 2001, ' "Like a possession of the devil": the diffusion of Nightingale nursing and Anglo-Australian relations', *International History of Nursing Journal*, 6, 2, pp. 52–8.

Goffman, E. 1963, *Stigma*, Englewood Cliffs, Prentice Hall.

Goldner, M. 2004, 'Consumption as activism: an examination of CAM as part of the consumer movement in health', in Tovey, P., Easthope, G. and Adams, J. (eds), *The Mainstreaming of Complementary and Alternative Medicine*, London, Routledge, pp. 11–24.

Gort, E.H. and Coburn, D. 1988, 'Naturopathy in Canada: changing relationships to medicine, chiropractic and the state', *Social Science & Medicine*, 26, 10, pp. 1061–72.

Grant Sarra Consultancy Services no date, 'Strategic Indigenous awareness: "to understand the present we must understand the past"', Launceston, Riawunna Centre for Aboriginal Education, University of Tasmania.

Gray, D. and Saggers, S. 2005, 'Indigenous health: the perpetuation of inequality', in Germov, J. (ed.), *Second Opinion: An Introduction to Health Sociology* (3rd edn), South Melbourne, Oxford University Press, pp. 111–28.

Gray, D.E. 2006, *Health Sociology: An Australian Perspective*, Frenchs Forest, Pearson Education.

Gregory, S. 2005, 'Living with chronic illness in the family setting', *Sociology of Health and Illness*, 27, 3, pp. 372–92.

Hammett, R.J.H. and Harris, R.D. 2002, 'Halting the growth in diagnostic testing', *Medical Journal of Australia*, 177, 3, pp. 124–5.

Hansen, E. 2007, 'CAM, wellness nursing and the new public health', in Adams, J. and Tovey, P. (eds), *Complementary and Alternative Medicine in Nursing and Midwifery: Towards a Critical Social Science*, London, Routledge.

Hansen, E. and Easthope, G. 2007, *Lifestyle in Medicine*, London, Routledge.

Hardey, M. 1999, 'Doctor in the house: the Internet as a source of lay health knowledge and the challenge to expertise', *Sociology of Health and Illness*, 21, 6, pp. 820–35.

Hardey, M. 2002, ' "The story of my illness": personal accounts of illness on the Internet', *Health: An Interdisciplinary Journal for the Social Study of Health, Illness and Medicine*, 6, 1, pp. 31–46.

Harrington, J.M. 2001, 'Health effects of shift work and extended hours of work', *Occupational and Environmental Medicine*, 58, pp. 68–72.

Harris, M. and Telfer, B. 2001, 'The health needs of asylum seekers living in the community', *Medical Journal of Australia*, 175, pp. 589–92.

Harrison, J. 1999, 'A lavender pink grey power: gay and lesbian gerontology in Australia', *Australasian Journal on Ageing*, 18, 1, pp. 32–7.

Harrison, J. 2005, 'Pink, lavender and grey: gay, lesbian, bisexual, transgender and intersex ageing in Australian gerontology', *Gay & Lesbian Issues and Psychology Review*, 1, 1, pp. 11–16.

Hazelton, M. 2004, 'Mental health, citizenship and human rights', in Grbich, C. (ed.), *Health in Australia: Sociological Concepts and Issues* (3rd edn), Frenchs Forest, Pearson Education, pp. 200–15.

Hegney, D., Eley, R., Buikstra, E., Rees, S. and Patterson, E. 2006, 'Consumers' level of comfort with an advanced practice role for registered nurses in general practice: a Queensland, Australia, study', *Australian Journal of Primary Health*, 12, 3, pp. 44–51.

Helman, C. 1978, ' "Feed a cold, starve a fever": folk models of infection in an English suburban community, and their relation to medical treatment', *Culture, Medicine & Psychiatry*, 2, pp. 107–37.

Henderson, A. 2006, 'The evolving relationship of technology and nursing practice: negotiating the provision of care in a high tech environment', *Contemporary Nurse*, 22, pp. 59–65.

Hillier, L. and Harrison, L. 1999, 'The girls in our town: sex, love, relationships and rural life', in La Nauze, H., Briskman, L. and Lynn, M. (eds), *Challenging Rural Practice: Human Services in Australia*, Melbourne, Australian Research Centre in Sex, Health & Society.

Hirschkorn, K. 2006, 'Exclusive versus everyday forms of professional knowledge: legitimacy claims in conventional and alternative medicine', *Sociology of Health and Illness*, 28, 5, pp. 533–57.

Ho, C. 2006, 'Women crossing borders: the changing identities of professional Chinese migrant women in Australia', *Journal of Multidisciplinary International Studies*, 3, 2, http://epress.lib.uts.edu.au/ojs/index.php/portal.

Hocking, B. 2003, 'Reducing mental illness, stigma and discrimination: everybody's business', *Medical Journal of Australia*, 178, 9, pp. 47–8.

Holmes, D., Hughes, K.P. and Julian, R. 2003, *Australian Society: A Changing Society*, Frenchs Forest, Pearson Education.

Hughner, R.S. and Kleine, S.S. 2004, 'Views of health in the lay sector: a compilation and review of how individuals think about health', *Health: An Inter-disciplinary Journal for the Social Study of Health, Illness and Medicine*, 8, 4, pp. 395–422.

Hugo, G. 2004, 'Australia's most recent immigrants', *Australian Census Analytic Program*, Adelaide, The University of Adelaide.

Hunter, E., Hall, W. and Spargo, R. 1991, *The Distribution and Correlates of Alcohol Consumption in a Remote Aboriginal Population*, Monograph No. 12, Sydney, National Drug and Alcohol Research Centre.

Hyden, L.C. and Sachs, L. 1998, 'Suffering, hope and diagnosis: on the negotiation of chronic fatigue syndrome', *Health*, 2, 2, pp. 175–93.

Illich, I. 1976, *Limits to Medicine: Medical Nemesis, the Expropriation of Health*, London, Boyars.

Indigenous Nursing Education Working Group 2002, *"getting em n keepin em"*, Canberra, Commonwealth Department of Health and Ageing, Office for Aboriginal and Torres Strait Islander Health.

International Council of Nurses 2007, 'Definition of Nursing', www://inc.ch/definition.htm, accessed 25 June 2007.

Internet World 2006, 'Internet world stats', www.internetworldstats.com, accessed 12 February 2007.

Irvine, R. 1999, 'Losing patients: health care consumers, power and sociocultural change', in Grbich, C. (ed.), *Health in Australia: Sociological Concepts and Issues* (2nd edn), Sydney, Longman, pp. 191–214.

Irvine, R. 2002, 'Fabricating "health consumers" in health care politics', in Henderson, S. and Petersen, A.R. (eds), *Consumering Health: The Commodification of Health Care*, London, Routledge, pp. 31–47.

Jackson, L.R. and Ward, J. 1999, 'Aboriginal health: why is reconciliation necessary?', *Medical Journal of Australia*, 170, pp. 437–40.

Johnson, C. 2002, 'Heteronormative citizenship and the politics of passing', *Sexualities*, 5, 3, pp. 317–36.

Johnston, E. QC 1991, 'Royal Commission into Aboriginal Deaths in Custody: National Report Volume 1', www.austlii.edu.au/au/special/rsjproject/rsjlibrary/rciadic/national/vol1/1.html, accessed 11 September 2006.

Joyce, K. 2005, 'Appealing images: magnetic resonance imaging and the production of authoritative knowledge', *Social Studies of Science*, 35, pp. 437–62.

Julian, R. 2005, 'Ethnicity, health and multiculturalism', in Germov, J. (ed.), *Second Opinion: An Introduction to Health Sociology* (3rd edn), South Melbourne, Oxford University Press, pp. 149–67.

Jutel, A. 2006, 'The emergence of overweight as a disease entity: measuring up normality', *Social Science & Medicine*, 63, pp. 2268–76.

Kao, H.-F.S., Reeder, F.M., Hsu, M.-T. and Cheng, S.-F. 2006, 'A Chinese view of the Western nursing metaparadigm', *Journal of Holistic Nursing*, 24, pp. 92–101.

Kaptchuk, T.J. and Eisenberg, D.M. 1998, 'The persuasive appeal of alternative medicines', *Annals of Internal Medicine*, 129, 12, pp. 1061–5.

Kavanagh, A.M. and Broom, D.M. 1998, 'Embodied risk: my body, myself?', *Social Science & Medicine*, 46, 3, pp. 437–44.

Kawachi, I. 2002, 'What is social epidemiology?', *Social Science & Medicine*, 54, pp. 1739–41.

Kawachi, I. and Conrad, P. 1996, 'Medicalization and the pharmacological treatment of blood pressure', in Davis, P. (ed.), *Contested Ground: Public Purpose and Private Interest in the Regulation of Prescription Drugs*, New York, Oxford University Press, pp. 26–41.

Kawachi, I., Subramanian, S.V. and Almeida-Filho, N. 2002, 'A glossary for health inequalities', *Journal of Epidemiology and Community Health*, 56, pp. 647–52.

Kelaher, M., Williams, G. and Manderson, L. 2001, 'Population characteristics, health and social issues among Filipinas in Queensland Australia', *Journal of Ethnic and Migration Studies*, 27, 1, pp. 101–14.

Keleher, H. 2003, 'Public health nursing in Australia: historically invisible', *International History of Nursing Journal*, 7, 3, pp. 50–5.

Keleher, H. 2004a, 'Promoting healthy ageing', in Keleher, H. and Murphy, B. (eds), *Understanding Health: A Determinants Approach*, South Melbourne, Oxford University Press, pp. 312–17.

Keleher, H. 2004b, 'Social exclusion', in Keleher, H. and Murphy, B. (eds), *Understanding Health: A Determinants Approach*, South Melbourne, Oxford University Press, pp. 246–51.

Keleher, H. and Murphy, B. 2004, 'Understanding health: an introduction', in Keleher, H. and Murphy, B. (eds), *Understanding Health: A Determinants Approach*, South Melbourne, Oxford University Press, pp. 3–8.

Kelly, M. and Field, D. 1996, 'Medical sociology, chronic illness and the body', *Sociology of Health and Illness*, 18, pp. 241–57.

Kelner, M., Wellman, B., Boon, H. and Welsh, S. 2004, 'Responses of established healthcare to the professionalisation of complementary and alternative medicine in Ontario', *Social Science & Medicine*, 59, pp. 915–30.

Khan, K.S. 2000, 'Public health priorities and the social determinants of health', in Coulter, A. and Ham, C. (eds), *The Global Challenge of Health Care Rationing*, Buckingham, Open University Press, pp. 74–85.

Kivits, J. 2004, 'Researching the "informed patient": the case of online health information seekers', *Information, Communication & Society*, 7, 4, pp. 510–30.

Kleinman, A. 1988, *The Illness Narratives: Suffering, Healing and the Human Condition*, New York, Basic Books.

Koutroulis, G. 1990, 'The orifice revisited: women in gynaecological texts', *Community Health Studies*, 14, 1, pp. 73–84.

Koutroulis, G. 2003, 'Detained asylum seekers, health care and questions of human(e)ness', *Australian and New Zealand Journal of Public Health*, 27, 4, pp. 381–4.

Kuhn, T.S. 1962, *The Structure of Scientific Revolutions*, Chicago, University of Chicago Press.

Kurz, P. 1994, 'The growth of antiscience', *Skeptical Inquirer*, 18, 3, pp. 225–63.

Langer, B. 2002, 'The consuming self', in Beilharz, P. and Hogan, T. (eds), *Social Self, Global Culture: An Introduction to Sociological Ideas* (2nd edn), South Melbourne, Oxford University Press, pp. 55–66.

Last, J.M. 1995, *A Dictionary of Epidemiology* (3rd edn), New York, Oxford University Press.

Laurant, M., Reeves, D., Hermens, R., Braspenning, J., Grol, R. and Sibbald, B. 2004, 'Substitution of doctors by nurses in primary care', *Cochrane Database Systematic Review*, 5, 4, Art no. CD001271. DOI: 10.1002/14651858.CD001271.pub2.

Lee, S. and Mysyk, A. 2004, 'The medicalisation of compulsive buying', *Social Science & Medicine*, 58, pp. 1709–18.

Leonard, W. 2002, 'Introductory paper: developing a framework for understanding patterns of health and illness specific to gay, lesbian, bisexual, transgender and intersex (GLBTI) people', in Leonard, W. (ed.), *What's the Difference? Health Issues of Major Concern to Gay, Lesbian, Bisexual, Transgender and Intersex (GLBTI) Victorians*, Melbourne, Ministerial Advisory Committee on Gay and Lesbian Health, Victorian Government Department of Human Services, pp. 3–12.

Lew-Ting, C.-Y. 2005, 'Antibiomedicine belief and integrative health seeking in Taiwan', *Social Science & Medicine*, 60, pp. 2111–16.

Lin, V. and Pearse, W. 1990, 'A workforce at risk', in Reid, J. and Trompf, P. (eds), *The Health of Immigrant Australia*, Sydney, Harcourt Brace Jovanavich.

Link, B.G. and Phelan, J.C. 2001, 'Conceptualising stigma', *Annual Review of Sociology*, 27, pp. 363–529.

Link, B.G. and Phelan, J.C. 2006, 'Stigma and its public health implications', *The Lancet*, 367, pp. 528–9.

Lippman, A. 1992, 'Led (astray) by genetic maps: the cartography of the human genome and health care', *Social Science & Medicine*, 35, 12, pp. 1469–76.

Lockyer, L. and Bury, M. 2002, 'The construction of a modern epidemic: the implications for women of the gendering of coronary heart disease', *Journal of Advanced Nursing*, 39, 5, pp. 432–40.

Lopez, R.A. 2005, 'Use of alternative folk medicine by Mexican American women', *Journal of Immigrant Health*, 7, 1, pp. 23–31.

Lowe, I. 1989, 'Choosing health care technologies', *New Doctor*, 51, pp. 10–13.

Lowenthal, R.M. 2005, 'Public illness: how the community recommended complementary and alternative medicine for a prominent politician with cancer', *Medical Journal of Australia*, 183, 11/12, pp. 576–9.

Loxton, D., Hussain, R. and Schofield, M. 2003, 'Women's experiences of domestic abuse in rural and remote Australia', 7th National Rural Health Conference, Hobart, Tasmania.

Lozano Applewhite, S. 1995, 'Curanderismo: demystifying the health beliefs and practices of elderly Mexican Americans', *Health and Social Work*, 20, 4, pp. 247–53.

Ludman, E.K., Newman, J.M. and Lynn, L.L. 1989, 'Blood-building foods in contemporary Chinese populations', *Journal of the American Dietetic Association*, 89, 8, pp. 1122–5.

Lupton, D. 1993, 'The construction of patienthood in medical advertising', *International Journal of Health Services*, 23, 4, pp. 805–19.

Lupton, D. 1998, 'Medicine and health care in the popular media', in Petersen, A.R. and Waddell, C. (eds), *Health Matters: Sociology of Health and Illness*, St Leonards, Allen & Unwin, pp. 194–207.

Lupton, D. 2003, *Medicine as Culture* (2nd edn), London, Sage Publications.

Lupton, D. 2005, 'The body, medicine and society', in Germov, J. (ed.), *Second Opinion: An Introduction to Health Sociology* (3rd edn), South Melbourne, Oxford University Press, pp. 195–207.

Lupton, D. and Chapman, S. 1994, 'Freaks, moral tales & medical marvels: health & medical stories on Australian television', *Media Information Australia*, 72, May, pp. 94–103.

Macdonald, J.J. 2006, 'Shifting paradigms: a social-determinants approach to solving problems in men's health policy and practice', *Medical Journal of Australia*, 185, 8, pp. 456–8.

MacDougall, C. 2003, 'Learning from differences between ordinary and expert theories of health and physical activity', *Critical Public Health*, 13, 4, pp. 381–97.

MacIntyre, S., Ford, G. and Hunt, K. 1999, 'Do women "over-report" morbidity? Men's and women's responses to structured prompting on a standard question on long standing illness', *Social Science & Medicine*, 48, 1, pp. 89–98.

MacKenzie, D. and Wajcman, J. 1999, 'Introductory essays: the social shaping of technology', in MacKenzie, D. and Wajcman, J. (eds), *The Social Shaping of Technology*, Maidenhead, Open University Press pp. 3–27.

MacLennan, A.H., Myers, S.P. and Taylor, A.W. 2006, 'The continuing use of complementary and alternative medicine in South Australia: costs and beliefs in 2004', *Medical Journal of Australia*, 184, 1, pp. 27–31.

Maher, P. 1999, 'A review of "traditional" Aboriginal health beliefs', *Australian Journal of Rural Health*, 7, 4, pp. 229–36.

Malone, R.E. 2003, 'Distal nursing', *Social Science & Medicine*, 56, pp. 2317–26.

Mathers, C., Vos, T. and Stevenson, C. 1999, *The Burden of Disease and Injury in Australia*, Canberra, Australian Institute of Health and Welfare.

Mathers, C.D. and Schofield, M. 1998, 'The health consequences of unemployment: the evidence', *Medical Journal of Australia*, 168, pp. 178–82.

May, C., Allison, G., Chapple, A., Chew-Graham, C., Dixon, C., Gask, L., Graham, R., Rogers, A. and Roland, M. 2004, 'Framing the doctor–patient relationship in chronic illness: a comparative study of general practitioner accounts', *Sociology of Health and Illness*, 26, 2, pp. 135–58.

May, C. and Sirur, D. 1998, 'Art, science and placebo: incorporating homeopathy in general practice', *Sociology of Health and Illness*, 20, 2, pp. 168–90.

McClean, S. 2005, ' "The illness is part of the person": discourses of blame, individual responsibility and individuation at a centre for spiritual healing in the north of England', *Sociology of Health and Illness*, 27, 5, pp. 628–48.

McKinlay, J. 1981, 'From "promising report" to "standard procedure": seven stages in the career of medical innovation', *Millbank Quarterly*, 59, 3, pp. 374–410.

McNair, R. and Harrison, J. 2002, 'Life stage issues within GLBTI communities', in Leonard, W. (ed.), *What's the Difference? Health Issues of Major Concern to Gay, Lesbian, Bisexual, Transgender and Intersex (GLBTI) Victorians*, Melbourne, Ministerial Advisory Committee on Gay and Lesbian Health, Victorian Government Department of Human Services, pp. 37–44.

McNair, R. and Medland, N. 2002, 'Physical health issues for GLBTI Victorians', in Leonard, W. (ed.), *What's the Difference? Health Issues of Major Concern to Gay, Lesbian, Bisexual, Transgender and Intersex (GLBTI) Victorians*, Melbourne, Victorian Government Department of Human Services, pp. 13–19.

Meeker, W.C. and Haldeman, S. 2002, 'Chiropractic: a profession at the crossroads of mainstream and alternative medicine', *Annals of Internal Medicine*, 136, 3, pp. 216–27.

Melville, A. and Johnson, C. 1982, *Cured to Death: The Effects of Prescription Drugs*, London, Angus and Robertson.

Miers, M. 1999, 'Nurses in the labour market: exploring and explaining nurses' work', in Wilkinson, G. and Miers, M. (eds), *Power and Nursing Practice*, London, Macmillan, pp. 83–96.

Milio, N. 1983, 'Commentary: next steps in community health policy: matching rhetoric and reality', *Community Health Studies*, V11, 2, pp. 185–92.

Mills, C.W. 1959, *The Sociological Imagination*, Middlesex, Harmondsworth.

Minas, I.H. and Sawyer, S.M. 2002, 'The mental health of immigrant and refugee children and adolescents', *Medical Journal of Australia*, 177, pp. 404–5.

Mission Australia 2004, 'Fact sheet poverty: children and young people in Australia', www.missionaustralia.com.au, accessed 15 September 2006.

Mission Australia 2005, 'The voices of homeless young Australians, snapshot 2005', www.missionaustralia.com.au, accessed 15 September 2006.

Montagne, M. 1996, 'The Pharmakon phenomenom: cultural conceptions of drugs and drugs use', in Davis, P. (ed.), *Contested Ground: Public Purpose and Private Interest in the Regulation of Prescription Drugs*, New York, Oxford University Press, pp. 11–25.

Moser, A., van der Bruggen, H. and Widdershoven, G. 2006, 'Competency in shaping one's life: autonomy of people with type 2 diabetes mellitus in a nurse-led, shared-care setting; a qualitative study', *International Journal of Nursing Studies*, 43, pp. 417–27.

Moynihan, R. and Cassels, A. 2005, *Selling Sickness: How Drug Companies Are Turning Us All Into Patients*, Crows Nest, Allen & Unwin.

Mulhall, A. 1996, *Epidemiology, Nursing and Healthcare*, London, Macmillan.

Murphy, K. and Stafford, A. 2006, 'Stem cell research gets green light', *The Age*, 8 November, www.theage.com.au/news/national/stem-cell-research-gets-green-light/2006/11/07/1162661685130.html, accessed 3 April 2007.

Murray, J. and Shepherd, S. 1993, 'Alternative or additional medicine? An exploratory study in general practice', *Social Science & Medicine*, 37, 8, pp. 983–8.

Myers, S.P. and Cheras, P.A. 2004, 'The other side of the coin: safety of complementary and alternative medicine', *Medical Journal of Australia*, 181, 4, pp. 222–5.

Najman, J. and Western, J. 2000, 'Introduction', in Najman, J. and Western, J. (eds), *A Sociology of Australian Society*, South Yarra, Macmillan.

National Aboriginal and Torres Strait Islander Health Council 2000, *National Aboriginal and Torres Strait Islander Health Strategy, Consultation draft*, Canberra, National Aboriginal and Torres Strait Islander Health Council.

National Aboriginal Health Strategy Working Party 1989, *A National Aboriginal Health Strategy*, Canberra, National Aboriginal Health Strategy Working Party.

National Nursing & Nursing Education Taskforce 2005, *Nurse Practitioners in Australia: Mapping of State/Territory Nurse Practitioner (NP) Models, Legislation and Authorisation Process*, Melbourne, National Nursing & Nursing Education Taskforce.

National Obesity Taskforce 2002, *Healthy Weight 2008. Australia's Future: The National Action Agenda for Young Children and Young People and their Families*, Canberra, Commonwealth of Australia.

Nelkin, D. 1991, 'AIDS and the news media', *Millbank Quarterly*, 69, pp. 293–307.

Nelson, S. 2001, 'Hairdressing and nursing', *Collegian*, 8, 2, pp. 28–31.

Nettleton, S. 1995, *The Sociology of Health and Illness*, Cambridge, Polity Press.

Nunkoosing, K. and Cook, K. 2006, '*I have had a past and I suppose I have a future but...' A report to the Aged and Community Care Team*, Melbourne, Brotherhood of St Laurence.

O'Donnell, S., Condell, S., Begley, C. and Fitzgerald, T. 2006, 'Prehospital care pathway delays: gender and myocardial infarction', *Journal of Advanced Nursing*, 53, 3, pp. 268–76.

O'Shaughnessy, M. and Stadler, J. 2005, *Media and Society: An Introduction* (3rd edn), South Melbourne, Oxford University Press.

Osborn, M. and Smith, J.A. 2006, 'Living with a body separate from the self. The experience of the body in chronic benign low back pain: an interpretive phenomenological analysis', *Scandinavian Journal of Caring Sciences*, 20, 2, pp. 216–28.

Panel on Definition and Description CRMCA1 1997, 'Defining and describing complementary and alternative medicine', *Alternative Therapies*, 3, pp. 49–57.

Parle, J., Ross, N. and Doe, W. 2006, 'The medical practitioner: developing a physician assistance equivalent for the United Kingdom', *Medical Journal of Australia*, 185, 1, pp. 13–17.

Parslow, R., Jorm, J., Christensen, H., Jacomb, P. and Rodgers, B. 2004, 'Gender differences in factors affecting use of health services: an analysis of a community study of middle-aged and older Australians', *Social Science & Medicine*, 59, pp. 2121–9.

Pascoe, T., Foley, E., Hutchinson, R., Watts, I., Whitecross, L. and Snowdon, T. 2005, 'The changing face of nurses in Australian general practice', *Australian Journal of Advanced Nursing*, 23, 1, pp. 44–50.

Patton, S. 2003, *Pathways: How Women Leave Violent Men*, Hobart, Women Tasmania, Department of Premier and Cabinet.

Petersen, A.R. 1994, *In a Critical Condition: Health and Power Relations in Australia*, St Leonards, Allen & Unwin.

Petersen, A.R. and Lupton, D. 1996, *The New Public Health: Health and Self in the Age of Risk*, St Leonards, Allen & Unwin.

Phelan, J.C., Link, B.G., Stueve, A. and Pescosolido 2000, 'Public conceptions of mental illness in 1960 and 1996: what is mental illness and is it to be feared?', *Journal of Health and Social Behaviour*, 41, 2, pp. 188–207.

Pill, R. 1991, 'Issues in lifestyles and health: lay meanings of health and health behaviour', in Badura, B. and Kickbusch, I. (eds), *Health Promotion Research: Towards a New Social Epidemiology*, Copenhagen, WHO Regional Publications, European Series, pp. 187–211.

Pinder, P. 1995, 'Bringing back the body without the blame?: the experience of ill and disabled people at work', *Sociology of Health and Illness*, 17, 5, pp. 605–31.

Pinell, P. 1996, 'Modern medicine and the civilising process', *Sociology of Health and Illness*, 18, 1, pp. 1–16.

Pitts, M., Smith, A., Mitchell, A. and Patel, S. 2006, *Private Lives: A Report on the Health and Wellbeing of GLBTI Australians*, Monograph Series No. 57, Melbourne, Australian Research Centre in Sex, Health and Society, La Trobe University.

Popay, J. and Williams, G. 1996, 'Public health research and lay knowledge', *Social Science & Medicine*, 42, 5, pp. 759–68.

Porter, S. 1997, 'Sociology and the nursing curriculum: a further comment', *Journal of Advanced Nursing*, 26, 1, pp. 214–18.

Porter, S. 1999, 'Working with doctors', in Wilkinson, G. and Miers, M. (eds), *Power and Nursing Practice*, London, Macmillan, pp. 97–110.

Prior, L. 2003, 'Belief, knowledge and expertise: the emergence of the lay expert in medical sociology', *Sociology of Health and Illness*, 25, pp. 41–57.

Productivity Commission 2005, *Australia's Health Workforce*, Research Report, Canberra, Productivity Commission.

Quinlan, M. and Bohle, P. 1991, *Managing Occupational Health and Safety in Australia: A Multidisciplinary Approach*, Crows Nest, Macmillan.

Reporters Without Borders 2006, 'Worldwide Press Freedom Index 2006', www.rsf.org, accessed 12 February 2007.

Reutter, L.I., Sword, W., Meagher-Stewart, D. and Rideout, E. 2004, 'Nursing students' beliefs about poverty and health', *Journal of Advanced Nursing*, 48, 3, pp. 299–309.

Richmond, K. and Savvy, P. 2005, 'In sight, in mind: mental health policy in the era of deinstitutionalisation', *Health Sociology Review*, 14, 3, pp. 215–29.

Roach-Anleu, S. 2005, 'The medicalisation of deviance', in Germov, J. (ed.), *Second Opinion: An Introduction to Health Sociology* (3rd edn), South Melbourne, Oxford University Press, pp. 168–74.

Roberston, J. 2003, 'Extending preimplantation genetic diagnosis: medical and non-medical uses', *Journal of Medical Ethics*, 29, 4, pp. 213–16.

Robotin, M.C. and Penman, A.G. 2006, 'Integrating complementary therapies into mainstream cancer care: which way forward?', *Medical Journal of Australia*, 185, 7, pp. 377–9.

Ross, B., Snasdell-Taylor, J., Cass, Y. and Azmi, S. 2005, 'Health financing in Australia: the objectives and players', *Occasional Papers: Health Financing Series Volume 1*, Canberra, Australian Government Department of Health and Aged Care.

Royal College of Nursing Australia 2003, *Nursing in General Practice: A Guide for the General Practice Team*, Canberra, Australian Government Department of Health and Ageing.

Runciman, W., Roughead, E., Semple, S. and Adams, R. 2003, 'Adverse drug events and medication errors in Australia', *International Journal for Quality in Health*, 15, 1, pp. i49–i59.

Sachs, L. 1995, 'Is there a pathology of prevention? The implications of visualising the invisible in screening programs', *Culture, Medicine & Psychiatry*, 19, pp. 503–25.

Saks, M. 2003, *Orthodox and Alternative Medicine*, London, Continuum.

Salstonall, R. 1993, 'Healthy bodies, social bodies: men's and women's concepts and practices of health in everyday life', *Social Science & Medicine*, 36, pp. 7–14.

Saunders, P. 2003, *Can Social Exclusion Provide a New Framework for Measuring Poverty?* Discussion Paper no. 127, Sydney, Social Policy Research Centre.

Scambler, G. and Hopkins, A. 1986, 'Being epileptic: coming to terms with stigma', *Sociology of Health and Illness*, 8, 1, pp. 26–43.

Scheper-Hughes, N. 2001, 'Bodies for sale: whole or in parts', *Body & Society*, 7, 2–3, pp. 1–8.

Schoenberg, N.E., Amey, C.H. and Coward, R.T. 1998, 'Stories of meaning: lay perspectives on the origin and management of non-insulin dependent diabetes mellitus among older women in the United States', *Social Science & Medicine*, 47, 12, pp. 211–25.

Schultz, J. 1994, *Not Just Another Business: Journalists, Citizens and the Media*, Leichardt, Pluto Press.

Schulz, B. 1991, *A Tapestry of Service: The Evolution of Nursing in Australia*, Melbourne, Churchill Livingstone.

Schulze, B. and Angermayer, M.C. 2003, 'Subjective experiences of stigma. A focus group study of schizophrenic patients, their relatives and mental health professionals', *Social Science & Medicine*, 56, pp. 299–312.

Seale, C. 2002, *Media & Health*, London, Sage Publications.

See, K.A., Lavercombe, P.S., Dillon, J. and Ginsberg, R. 2006, 'Accidental death from acute selenium poisoning', *Medical Journal of Australia*, 185, 7, pp. 388–9.

Sen, A. 2000, *Social Exclusion: Concept Application and Scrutiny, Social Development*, Social Development Papers no. 1, Office of Environment and Social Development, Manila, Asia Development Bank.

Shaw, I. 2002, 'How lay are lay beliefs?', *Health: An Interdisciplinary Journal for the Social Study of Health, Illness and Medicine*, 6, 3, pp. 287–99.

Shiel, E. 1999, 'Don't ask for an opinion: ask for the scalpel: media coverage of breast cancer in Australia in 1995', Sydney, NHMRC National Breast Cancer Centre.

Shilling, C. 1993, *The Body and Social Theory*, London, Sage Publications.

Short, S.D. 2004, 'Fat is a fairness issue', in Schultz, J. (ed.), *Griffith Review 4: Making Perfect Bodies*, Sydney, ABC Books.

Short, S.D., Sharman, E. and Speedy, S. 1993, *Sociology for Nurses: An Australian Introduction*, South Melbourne, Macmillan.

Siahpush, M. 1998, 'Postmodern values, dissatisfaction with conventional medicine and popularity of alternative therapies', *Journal of Sociology*, 34, 1, pp. 58–70.

Singh, I. 2004, 'Doing their jobs: mothering with Ritalin in a culture of mother-blame', *Social Science & Medicine*, 59, pp. 1193–205.

Sirois, F.M. and Gick, M.L. 2002, 'An investigation of the health beliefs and motivations of complementary medicine clients', *Social Science & Medicine*, 55, pp. 1025–37.

Smith, J.D. 2004, *Australia's Rural and Remote Health: A Social Justice Perspective*, Croydon, Tertiary Press.

Smith Maguire, J. 2002, 'Body lessons: fitness publishing and the cultural production of the fitness consumer', *International Review for the Sociology of Sport*, 37, 3–4, pp. 449–64.

Sontag, S. 1991, *Illness as Metaphor and AIDS and its Metaphors*, London, Penguin.

Spitzack, C. 1992, 'Foucault's political body in medical praxis', in Leder, D. (ed.), *The Body in Medical Thought and Practice*, Dordrecht, Kluwer Academic, pp. 51–68.

Stacey, M. 1994, 'The power of lay knowledge: a personal view', in Popay, J. and Williams, G. (eds), *Researching the People's Health*, London, Routledge, pp. 85–98.

Standing Committee on Aboriginal and Torres Strait Islander Health 2002, *Aboriginal and Torres Strait Islander Health Workforce National Strategic Framework*, Canberra, AHMAC.

Standing Committee on Aboriginal and Torres Strait Islander Health and Statistical Information Management Committee 2006, *National Summary of the 2003 and 2004 Jurisdictional Reports against the Aboriginal and Torres Strait Islander Health Performance Indicators*. AIHW cat. no. IHW 16, Canberra, Australian Institute of Health and Welfare.

Stein, L. 1967, 'The doctor–nurse game', *Archives of General Psychiatry*, 16, pp. 699–703.

Stevens, M. 2006, 'Howard rescues Gardisil from Abbott's poison pill', *The Australian*, 11 November, www.theaustralian.news.com.au/story/0,20867,20736508-5001641,00.html, accessed 3 April 2007.

Stockdale, A. 1999, 'Waiting for the cure: mapping the social relations of human gene therapy research', *Sociology of Health and Illness*, 21, 5, pp. 579–96.

Strauss, A. 1981, 'Chronic illness', in Conrad, P. and Kern, R. (eds), *The Sociology of Health and Illness: Critical Perspectives*, New York, St Martin's Press, pp. 138–49.

Strazdins, L. and Bammer, G. 2004, 'Women, work and musculoskeletal health', *Social Science & Medicine*, 58, 6, pp. 997–1005.

Strazzari, M. 2006, 'Ageing, dying and death in the twenty-first century', in Germov, J. (ed.), *Second Opinion: An Introduction to Health Sociology* (3rd edn), South Melbourne, Oxford University Press, pp. 244–64.

Sultan, A. and O'Sullivan, K. 2001, 'Psychological disturbances in asylum seekers held in long term detention: a participant–observer account', *Medical Journal of Australia*, 175, pp. 593–6.

Svensson, R. 1996, 'The interplay between doctors and nurses: a negotiated perspective', *Sociology of Health and Illness*, 18, 3, pp. 379–98.

Taylor, S.D. 2004, 'Predictive genetic test decisions for Huntington's disease: context, appraisal and new moral imperatives', *Social Science & Medicine*, 58, pp. 137–49.

Taylor, S.E. 1979, 'Hospital patient behaviour: reactance, helplessness or control?', *Journal of Social Issues*, 35, 1, pp. 156–84.

Thomson, N. 2003, 'The need for Indigenous health information', in Thomson, N. (ed.), *The Health of Indigenous Australians*, South Melbourne, Oxford University Press, pp. 1–24.

Tovey, P. and Adams, J. 2003, 'Nostalgic and nostophobic referencing and the authentication of nurses' use of complementary therapies', *Social Science & Medicine*, 56, pp. 1469–80.

Tovey, P., Easthope, G. and Adams, J. 2004, *The Mainstreaming of Complementary and Alternative Medicine: Studies in Social Context*, London, Routledge.

Trewin, D. and Madden, R. 2005, *The Health and Welfare of Australia's Aboriginal and Torres Strait Islander Peoples*. ABS cat. no. 4704.0, AIHW cat. no. IHW14, Canberra, Australian Bureau of Statistics and Australian Institute of Health and Welfare.

Trostle, J.A. 1988, 'Medical compliance as an ideology', *Social Science & Medicine*, 27, 12, pp. 1299–308.

Turner, B.S. 1987, *Medical Power and Social Knowledge*, Beverly Hills, Sage.

Turner, B.S. 2004, 'Foreword: the end(s) of scientific medicine?', in Tovey, P., Easthope, G. and Adams, J. (eds), *The Mainstreaming of Complementary and Alternative Medicine: Studies in Social Context*, London, Routledge, pp. xiii–xx.

Turrell, G., Stanley, L., de Looper, M. and Oldenburg, B. 2006, *Health Inequalities in Australia: Morbidity, Health Behaviours, Risk Factors and Health Service Use.*, Health Inequalities Monitoring Series No. 2. AIHW cat. no. PHE 72, Canberra, Queensland Institute of Technology and the Australian Institute of Health and Welfare.

University Department of Rural Health, Indigenous Health Website, University of Tasmania, www.ruralhealth.utas.edu.au/indigenous-health/

Van Krieken, R., Habibis, D., Smith, P., Hutchins, B., Haralambos, M. and Holborn, M. 2006, *Sociology: Themes and Perspectives* (3rd edition), Frenchs Forest, Pearson Education Australia.

Van Krieken, R., Smith, P., Habibis, D., McDonald, K., Haralambos, M. and Holborn, M. 2000, *Sociology: Themes and Perspectives* (2nd edition), Frenchs Forest, Pearson Education.

Victorian Gay and Lesbian Rights Lobby 2000, *Enough is Enough: A Report on the Discrimination and Abuse Experienced by Lesbians, Gay Men, Bisexuals and Transgender People in Victoria*, Melbourne, Victorian Gay and Lesbian Rights Lobby.

Vincent, J.A. 2006, 'Ageing contested: anti-ageing science and the cultural construction of old age', *Sociology*, 40, 4, pp. 681–98.

Wainer, J. and Chesters, J. 2000, 'Rural mental health: neither romanticism nor despair', *Australian Journal of Rural Health*, 8, pp. 141–7.

Waitzkin, H. 1979, 'A Marxian interpretation of the growth and development of coronary care technology', *American Journal of Public Health*, 69, 12, pp. 1260–8.

Warburton, J. and McLaughlin, D. 2005, '"Lots of little kindness": valuing the role of older Australians as informal volunteers in the community', *Ageing & Society*, 25, pp. 715–30.

Waters, M. and Crook, R. 1993, *Sociology One: Principles of Sociological Analysis for Australians* (3rd edn), Melbourne, Longman Cheshire.

Watts, I., Foley, E., Hutchinson, R., Pascoe, T., Whitecross, L. and Snowdon, T. 2004, 'General practice nursing in Australia', Canberra, Royal Australian College of General Practitioners.

Wearing, B. 1996, *Gender: The Pain and Pleasure of Difference*, Melbourne, Longman.

Wearing, M. 2004, 'Medical dominance and the division of labour in the health professions', in Grbich, C. (ed.), *Health in Australia: Sociological Concepts and Issues*, Frenchs Forest, Pearson Education Australia, pp. 260–89.

Weber, M. 1964, *The Theory of Social and Economic Organisation*, New York, Free Press.

Webster, A. 2002, 'Innovative health technologies and the social: redefining health, medicine and the body', *Current Sociology*, 50, 3, pp. 443–57.

Weiss, G.L. and Lonnquist, L.E. 2006, *The Sociology of Health, Healing, and Illness*, New Jersey, Pearson Prentice Hall.

Weitz, R. 2004, *The Sociology of Health, Illness and Health Care: A Critical Approach*, Southbank, Thomson Wadsworth.

Welsh, S., Kelner, M., Wellman, B. and Boon, H. 2004, 'Moving forward? Complementary and alternative practitioners seeking self regulation', *Sociology of Health and Illness*, 26, 2, pp. 216–41.

Werner, A. and Maltrud, K. 2003, 'It is hard work behaving as a credible patient: encounters between women with chronic pain and their doctors', *Social Science & Medicine*, 57, pp. 1409–19.

White, K. 1991, 'The sociology of health & illness: a trend report', *Current Sociology*, 39, 2, pp. 1–125.

Whitehead, L. 2006, 'Quest, chaos and restitution: living with chronic fatigue syndrome/ myalgic encephalomyelitis', *Social Science & Medicine*, 62, pp. 2236–45.

Wicks, D. 2005, 'Nursing and sociology: an uneasy relationship', in Germov, J. (ed.), *Second Opinion: An Introduction to Health Sociology*, South Melbourne, Oxford University Press, pp. 314–31.

Wiles, R. 1998, 'Patients' perceptions of their heart attack and recovery: the influence of epidemiological "evidence" and personal experience', *Social Science & Medicine*, 46, 11, pp. 1477–86.

Wilkinson, G. and Miers, M. 1999, 'Power and professions', in Wilkinson, G. and Miers, M. (eds), *Power and Nursing Practice*, London, Macmillan, pp. 24–36.

Wilkinson, R.G., Kawachi, I. and Kennedy, B.P. 1998, 'Mortality, the social environment, crime and violence', in Bartley, M., Blane, D. and Davey Smith, G. (eds), *The Sociology of Health Inequalities*, Oxford, Blackwell, pp. 19–38.

Williams, C. 2000, 'Doing health, doing gender: teenagers, diabetes and asthma', *Social Science & Medicine*, 50, pp. 387–96.

Williams, C., Cooke, H. and May, C. 1998, *Sociology, Nursing and Health*, Oxford, Butterworth-Heinemann.

Williams, S. 1987, 'Goffman, interactionism and the management of stigma in everyday life', in Scambler, G. (ed.), *Sociological Theory & Medical Sociology*, London, Tavistock.

Williams, S. 2000, 'Chronic illness as biographical disruption or biographical disruption as a chronic illness? Reflection on a core concept', *Sociology of Health and Illness*, 22, 1, pp. 40–67.

Williamson, G.R. 1999, 'Teaching sociology to nurses: exploring the debate', *Journal of Clinical Nursing*, 8, pp. 269–74.

Willis, E. 1989, *Medical Dominance* (revised edn), St Leonards, Allen & Unwin.

Willis, E. 1994, *Illness and Social Relations: Issues in the Sociology of Health Care*, St Leonards, Allen & Unwin.

Willis, E. 1995, 'The political economy of genes', *Journal of Australian Political Economy*, 36, pp. 104–13.

Willis, E. 1998, 'The "new" genetics and the sociology of medical technology', *Journal of Sociology*, 34, 2, pp. 170–83.

Willis, K. and Baxter, J. 2003, 'Trusting technology: women aged 40–49 years participating in screening for breast cancer: an exploratory study', *Australian and New Zealand Journal of Public Health*, 27, 3, pp. 282–6.

Wilson, K., Coulon, L., Hillege, S. and Swann, W. 2005, 'Nurse practitioners' experiences of working collaboratively with general practitioners and allied health professionals in New South Wales, Australia', *Australian Journal of Advanced Nursing*, 23, 2, pp. 22–7.

Wiseman, J. 1998, *Global Nation? Australia and the Politics of Globalization*, Melbourne, Cambridge University Press.

Witz, A. 1992, *Professions and Patriarchy*, London, Routledge.

World Health Organization 1948, 'Health is a state of complete physical, mental and social well-being and not merely the absence of disease or infirmity.' Preamble to the Constitution of the World Health Organization as adopted by the International Health Conference, New York, 19–22 June, 1946; signed on 22 July 1946 by the representatives of 61 States (Official Records of the World Health Organization, no. 2, p. 100) and entered into force on 7 April 1948, New York, World Health Organization.

World Health Organization 1976, *Definition of Disability*, Document A29/INFDOVI/1, Geneva, World Health Organization.

Wynne, B. 1996, 'May the sheep safely graze? A reflexive view of the expert–lay knowledge divide', in Lash, S., Szerszynski, B. and Wynne, B. (eds), *Risk, Environment and Modernity: Towards a New Ecology*, London, Sage, pp. 44–83.

Young, C. 1992, 'Mortality, the ultimate indicator of survival: the differential experience between birthplace groups', in Donovan, J., d'Espaignet, E.T., Merton, C. and van Ommeren, M. (eds), *Immigrants in Australia: A Health Profile*, Canberra, AGPS.

Young, I.M. 1990, *Throwing Like a Girl and Other Essays in Feminist Philosophy and Social Theory*, Bloomington, Indiana University Press.

Zadoroznyj, M. 1998, 'Transformation in collective identity of nurses', in Keleher, H. and McInerney, F. (eds), *Nursing Matters: Critical Sociological Perspectives*, Marrickville, Churchill Livingstone.

Zadoroznyj, M. 2004, 'Gender and health', in Grbich, C. (ed.), *Health in Australia: Sociological Concepts and Issues*, Frenchs Forest, Pearson Longman, pp. 128–50.

Zeiler, K. 2004, 'Reproductive autonomous choice: a cherished illusion? Reproductive autonomy examined in the context of preimplantation genetic diagnosis', *Medicine, Health Care and Philosophy*, 7, 2, pp. 175–83.

Zollman, C. and Vickers, A. 1999, 'Users and practitioners of complementary medicine', *British Medical Journal*, 319, pp. 836–8.

index